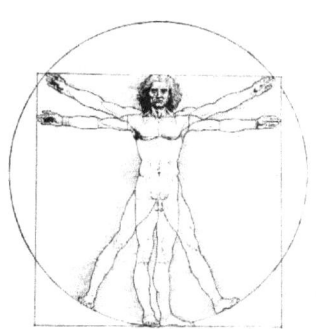

Tibetan Fusion

of Meditative Movement

Special thanks to all of the meditative movement teachers.

Introduction to Fusion

Tibetan Fusion is a combination of meditative movements to build your chi, your prana, your balanced life energy and an exploration of meditation. The simple movements are powerful on their own and integrate easily to form a highly effective practice to build balanced life energy. The primal meditative movements are comparable to the least common denominators in fraction problems, they are integrative and lead to the solution; balanced energy. Tibetan Fusion is composed of simple meditative movements, all akin to least common denominators, each easily accessible and beneficial to all.

Meditative movements are simply body movements, which no matter how physical, also develop the mind in their complexity and stimulate spirituality in their primal divinity. Meditative movements expend energy and at the same time attain it, increase relaxation and at the same time enhance awareness. On an analytical level the movements activate our potential in integrating the sympathetic (conscious) and parasympathetic (unconscious) aspects of the nervous system. Physically, meditative movements activate the secondary or inactive side of the body, stimulating balance and potentially instigating consciousness and recognition of unconsciousness. Metaphysically, meditative movements integrate mind, body and spirit, manifesting numerous benefits.

I've studied many different meditative movements and not one of my teachers learned, taught or practiced just one type of meditative movement. Despite their primary focus the yogis, martial artists and internal artists I learned from all integrated many forms into their practice. Not one of my teachers ever suggested to only practice one form or not to practice a particular form. Most of them literally advised to do it all. All of my teachers insisted that one should be mindful about how you practice and exactly what you include in your practice, but none suggested setting limitations to merely one theory and practice. In fact, the more experienced teachers applied fewer labels and involved less strict forms, as if they had gone full circle beginning with simple practices, gaining complex comprehension and ultimately returning to simple practices again. Many masterful teachers concentrate more on simplicity for in life simplicity tends to be beautiful and in meditative movement simplicity tends to be powerful as well as accessible.

"I fear not the man who has practiced 10,000 kicks once, but I fear the man who has practiced one kick 10,000 times." ~Bruce Lee

Simplicity leads to mastery, not to mediocrity. To focus on practicing one simple kick is to approach mastery. Immersion in one system of yoga, or only practicing one form of tai chi will alone provide physical, mental and spiritual reward and perhaps mastery, but the road can be long and often revolves back to practicing the simpler starting points, the common denominators. Different practices are basically systems of 10,000 kicks. Practice and refinement of just a few of the simplest kicks from various systems of 10,000 kicks can be very rewarding and powerful enough to frighten the likes of Bruce Lee. Mastery of simple practices leads to more heightened understanding of complexity too for complex movements are more often just variations of simpler ones. Combination of simple practices can offer opportunity for development and enhancement for one's focus on practice is more important than the complexity of it. Meditative movements can be easy to learn, but their mastery is a never ending process.

Adopting and immersing oneself into one solitary practice is like only drinking orange juice. There is nothing wrong with that, in fact it's great. Only sometimes grapefruit juice is desirable and sometimes it's fun to have a variety of juices in a smoothie. Some say that some meditative movements, systems of 10,000 kicks, are complete practices and that there is no reason to attempt to add to a full glass so as to just dilute the drink. And yet if you add goodness to goodness you are left with goodness. Some say that it is better to dig one deep well than it is to dig many shallow holes. And yet in some environments if you know where you're digging you need not to dig deep before reaching plentiful spring water and all wells require many tools to construct and implement after all.

It is better to fuse simplicity than not to practice at all because of a perceived complex preventative. Sometimes the idea of digging a deep well in order to learn a series of meditative movements can be an intimidating process making many back away. Simple meditative movements can be more immediately compelling and lead to quantifiable and noticeable reward. And simple meditative movements constantly reveal subtleties despite being easy to learn. Simplicity combines well with simplicity and is adaptable to complexity. Combining complex flavors or complex meditative movements together might result in a funky taste or discomfort, but simple and primal meditative movements practically always go well together just as simple fruits practically always go well together.

Today the world is distracting and we are easily distracted. Today we lead different lives with different opportunities than we did even a decade ago. We live complex lives with analytical minds and mediated thoughts which compel us to have a hurried mind focusing on the tangible. But no matter how complex we have allowed society to become underneath it all we all seek simplicity, mostly believing it cannot be obtained without complexity. In fact, it is simple to be simple and completely up to you. Practicing meditation is simple and redirects our focus inward on intangible energy and insight.

Simple meditative movements maintain their primal compatibility providing access to balanced energy and with it relaxed awareness and grounded lightness. Meditative movements can be very much like a vacation away from complexity we can take at any time without any complex preparation. Sometimes the addition of one simple process can change or enhance what was considered complete recipe. Meditative movements are for many things, including strengthening and healing for instance and sometimes a small additive can assist these processes and enhance their overall applicability as practice for real life.

Today we spend an enormous time on computers to the point we do not pay attention to anything else, often communicating with each other through typing. Combined with all the other repetitive hand movements we often will have weakened and even arthritic hands. One exercise with martial roots also offers healing results to counter this predicament. Extend your hands in front of you and flick your fingers open from off of your thumb. Try to repeat 21 times each and go from there. Then extend your hands to your sides and flick open in the same manner. Then reach them above your head and flick open again in the same manner, an equal number of times. Be mindful not to lock your elbows or shoulders and to approach balance. This helps release tension in the hands, arms, shoulders and neck. It is simple and highly effective for alleviating tension, instigating healing and increasing strength. It is simple and beneficial on its own and is also an excellent warming preparation for the first movement of the Five Tibetan Rites of Rejuvenation, originally brought to the West by Peter Kelder. Try its integration.

Tibetan Fusion is like a mixture of fruits put together in quantities and qualities in accordance with overall gastronomical sensibility. The meditative movements are combined in the following order to allow anyone to increase their open access to balanced energy. And yet as part of being open one can utilize aspects of Tibetan Fusion however. Energy is like water and we are each like riverbeds, moving and flowing in different directions and currents. Each individual component in Tibetan Fusion can be done on its own or left out of the routine. Part of the power of meditative movement, simple or otherwise, is relaxed repetition, like stirring ingredients together or like creating static electricity. Most people are intimidated by complexity and bored by repetition which is more essential to meditative movement than complexity, so do not drop a practice simply because you learn it, make it practice.

Tibetan Fusion is a combines lying and standing asanas, chi gung energy movement, various squats, standing breathing practices, and The Five Tibetan Rites of Rejuvenation. Each of the movements are easy to learn and make your own, but require practice to master and refine. All systems of 10,000 kicks include various meditations or suggest integrating meditation to hone one's practice. Included is a thorough explanation of meditation, so as to simplify and demystify it. I learned various tai chi, chi gung, yoga, and different meditations and present correlating concepts from them to explain meditation. Tibetan Fusion provides information on balancing energy for beginners and longtime practitioners.

I practiced The Five Tibetan Rites of Rejuvenation for about 18 years and find that by itself it's extremely powerful. I also practiced various tai chi, chi gung and yoga and found The Five Tibetans can be enhanced or made more enjoyable with a few simple additions. In practicing different forms of meditative movement I noticed there are certain elements each has similarly and certain benefits each provide differently. Each practice operates as a vehicle if you will, each with its own way to get you to your destination. And just like you can't fly from your home to your hotel, just like you must take a boat or drive or hike occasionally, different vehicles are useful at different times on different points on the journey. Many vehicles are used for physical movement and many vehicles can be used in meditative movement as well. As long as one is mindful about where one is going and when one should take different vehicles they all work perfectly well together. In a meditative journey the same is applicable, as long as you are mindful of where you are going and of the adjustment of your mind state different vehicles work perfectly together. One's mind state should basically be seeking betterment of self in order to compassionately assist those around you and your surroundings. With devotion to this mind state you will benefit quickly from your practice and be able to follow through on taking compassionate integrative action in real life.

There are certain elements to meditative movement which are best done in a certain fashion or optimally done in a certain order, (tai chi practitioners frequently do lying and standing asanas before practicing breathing and the long form for instance) and if the ingredients are kept simple, to the point of being primal, they will mix well almost without question. There are certain dynamics to keep in mind, certain physical and mental rules to follow, but as long as you keep it simple, combining meditative movement works well and can even be superior to say only practicing one form of 10,000 kicks. Sometimes a simple variation or new addition in accordance to primal principles can be an inspiration and implement ascension.

No matter how complex a system of 10,000 kicks may be, the first few kicks are the most important in order to learn further and because the simple fundamentals also tend to be the most powerful. The Pareto Principle is frequently applied to economic subjects, but was originally derived from noticing that about 80% of a garden's harvest was from about 20% of the plants. In business it is reflected in the idea that 20% of clients bring 80% of business or 80% of your transactions occur during 20% of the calendar year. In martial and internal arts the Pareto Principle is applicable in the sense that the simplest 20% of your practice results in 80% of the reward. Tibetan Fusion is a combination of some of the 20% of various systems of 10,000 kicks. The fusion results in a rewarding practice you can easily integrate and make your own.

Fusion leads to strength. Humanity itself is a fusion and integration. No matter how proud one might be of racial, national, religious or cultural origins, today most all people are fusions. Powerful individuals are not perfect, they practice fusion; acceptance, integration and transmutation of weakness into strength. Weakness is expressed in rejecting potential and actual. The superiority of fusion is biologically illustrated in what is known as hybrid vigor. Hybrid vigor occurs more often than not when different plants and animals breed to produce a hybrid adopting the stronger traits of each parent.

Socially speaking there are innumerable ways we are all a fusion, socially and biologically. Fusion is not the opposite of purity, but the acceptance of totality. Acceptance leads to openness and strength. Fusion equates to the rare and sought after feeling of balance. Fusion is union and oneness.

"Purity must be achieved by an indivisible unity of method and wisdom..." ~14th Dalai Lama

Buddha and Tummo

Tibet is a land of confluence, a land of intermingling cultures and integrating ideas. The word tantra signifies such confluence and integration, fusion. It is Sanskrit for loom, a device which weaves together string into cloth and was variously used to describe the knots of string weaved together in a rug and the cord sacred mala bead necklaces were strung. Malas are prayer necklaces of 108 beads to assist mentally or vocally repeating a mantra 108 times. Tantra is an old word from an ancient language with many properties and uses. Today it is often used in reference to the union of lovemaking. It notes a mutually accepted connection, a tied knot of intertwined being, like lovemaking, but not necessarily beginning with or limited to.

Tantra is an ancient spiritual philosophy preceding Buddhism and Hinduism. The ideas unify the macrocosm with the microcosm, the universal and the individual, the feminine and the masculine, it representing integration. Tantra can refer to integrative knowledge and its continuation and building through a teacher or guru to student, signifying union and fusion; the acceptance, integration and transmutation of knowledge, like the string of life. Tantra is essentially spiritual knowledge of individuation and connection and should not be confused with merely yoga, just as yoga should not be confused with being simply asanas or physical postures. Tantric ideas and yoga practices are physical, but they are more metaphysical.

Humanity itself is a tantra; a fused weaving knot. Tantra should not be confused with yantra yoga from Tibet, or yantras, sacred symbolism. Yantra yoga is one of the oldest forms of yoga and because of the environmentally foreboding nature of Tibet and the varying secretive cultures of most meditative movements it is said to be one of the purest and least altered forms of yoga. Yantra yoga concentrates on moving into and out of asanas with the breath, as opposed to being in a position for multiple breaths. Tantra is the integration of yantra (philosophy, visual symbol) mantra (oral communication) and mudra, (physical positioning) each important aspects of yoga and life. In the past a teacher or guru was a requirement for instruction, today there are not enough gurus relative to those who require instruction, but there also more ways to learn more practices than ever.

The difference between a teacher and a guru is that gurus are so profound that merely being in their presence imparts answers without questioning, comfort and even bliss. A guru has the ability to teach and share spiritual and meditative knowledge, but also has the power to transmit comforting presence. Ideally we would all have gurus, not so that we know what path to follow, so that we know where we are going as we proceed on our own path, so that we can become powerful individuals on our own.

Today in Tibet and the rest of the world, the number of empowered individuals, the number of teachers and gurus, is eclipsed by the number of institutionalized individuals. The institutionalized greatly outnumber the individuated, most of us are under the thumb of authorities busy tending to survival rather than seeking individuation with the assistance of a teacher or guru. Tibet's gurus have been overwhelmed, engulfed and scattered by repressive authorities, the worldly ways of national and cultural institutions and the global submission to them. The gurus of Tibet, in the same way as gurus of most of the world, have been run off and eliminated, most recently and perhaps most starkly in Tibet.

Tibet is one of many places to be occupied by force, but the forceful institutionalization of such a profoundly spiritual nation like Tibet is a horror revelatory of how low the global collective of humanity has sunk. The indigenous Tibetans have undergone forceful gentrification and destruction as is typical for institutional takeover. The Chinese institutions are dominating and destroying the Tibetan culture of monastic mountain retreat and individuals around the world have allowed the apartheid like rule of Tibet to happen without catalyzed boycott of China or proactive political strategy. Allowing one of the most spiritual and compassionate nations to ever exist is a sad example of the postmodern collective gone astray, worldlings lacking gurus, hungry and distracted institutionalized people.

Institutions and individuals immersed in worldly ways ought to assist those who seek to live concentrating on spiritual development. This was the way of Tibetan culture, everyone supported the monastic. Today in China there is rampant religious repression of Tibetan Buddhism, and Falun Gong and Christianity and likely any organization that officials see as a potential threat or outlet for a threat to their hierarchy. Such religious and cultural repression stems from the fact that devotion leads to individuation, individual empowerment and ultimately empowerment of the collective.

Institutions, like China, would like to keep everyone controlled, quiet and unaware of their potential. Many martial arts have been changed similarly so as to not allow people to develop their fighting ability sure, but to prevent them from gaining the potential metaphysical understanding as well. Tai chi, for instance has many times been transformed from an internal/martial (metaphysical) art to simple exercise to reduce the results and to hide its potential. Devoted practice leads to individuation, the opposite of institutionalization.

China recently enacted laws essentially taking over Tibetan Buddhist monasteries instituting government officials at the few remaining monasteries. China also recently enacted a law attempting to limit Tibetan Buddhist reincarnation without government permission. China killed countless Tibetans, destroyed thousands of monasteries and has remade the nation of Tibet as theirs. Some Tibetans, cornered by rigid oppression, have resorted to self-immolation in order to call attention to the corruption and gentrification, the most such desperate protest in modern history. Many have set themselves on fire to raise awareness of their exploitation and cultural elimination.

Tibet is a land of indigenous integration, the mountainous crossroads of Asia. Tibet was a spiritual nation, one of tantra and sharing where many spent their entire lives dedicated to the spiritual journey and those around them supported them. This contrasts most of society that selfishly pursues materialistic goals. Assisting the spiritual development of others let alone following one's own spiritual path are not primary considerations for most people, throughout most of the world today.

The Dalai Lama, (Ocean Wisdom Guru) the spiritual leader of Tibet is chosen or rather found through spiritual predictions and tests concerning a person's lineage, not through heritage, but through reincarnation. The current Dalai Lama is the 14th reincarnation of a great spiritual teacher. Despite losing his homeland and despite his people being dispersed and worse, the Dalai Lama remains positive for even though Tibetan Buddhism is being restricted in Tibet it has been freed to the world.

The idea of an ocean guru might be at first confusing especially from the mountains of Tibet however the ocean symbolizes consciousness, the ethereal force everywhere, of which we are but a drop, though within us is an ocean unto ourselves. The idea also reminds me of aspects of many meditations, Buddhist and otherwise, where one imagines being a conduit of compassion, ultimately visualizing that compassionate energy eventually crossing the oceans. One way I learned this is to meditate and imagine that your loving presence emanates and extends across the oceans. Begin with imagining removing suffering and instilling happiness to all sentient beings thirty miles beyond you, then three hundred, then throughout your continent, then across the ocean nearest you, then all oceans and then the whole world. In order to really benefit from any meditation and meditative movement it's important to include such compassionate thinking in your practice.

In Tibet and across much of Asia reincarnation is considered to be fact that science cannot yet explain, a simple process of evolution. There are numerous instances of children knowing information which could indeed be explained in no other way but reincarnation and remembering past life experience or some other extraordinary psychic powers. Locating the next reincarnation of the Dalai Lama always requires psychic predictions of sorts. No other nation in the world upheld such spiritual transition of power in modern times, or perhaps ever. Most all national institutions keep power in the family or another form of oligarchy rather through spiritual transition.

Almost all national institutions act to maintain and obtain power resulting in war states, buffer states and ever changing borders. Nations frequently act out of fear of loss as well as on potential gains. China took over Tibet when England left India and Tibet no longer was useful as a buffer state. Until then Tibetans walked or rode horses wherever they went, following a prophecy which stated that when the wheel comes to Tibet the nation would fall. China took over Tibet like so many other nations have taken over so many other spiritual places, like England took over India and like the European nations took over the entire world over centuries of colonialism.

Tibet is a place of mountain isolation and alternatively a place of integration at the crossroads, where it's said your hand in the sun can burn while your other hand in the shade is frost bitten. Great Indian gurus travelled to China via Tibet and likewise great Chinese philosophers and physicians went to India via Tibet. Even the legendary Mongolian armies came to Tibet as did people from the Muslim world and throughout Asia. Tibet is the Himalayan roof of the world and to a large extent it was the middle of the ancient world.

When Buddhism reached the Himalayan Mountains of Tibet from India it was integrated with ideas in the shamanistic Bonn religion, the prominent form of worship in Tibet. In Tibet the indigenous Bonn ideas, Buddhism, some Hindu beliefs, some Taoist and Chinese influences and other cultural philosophies were all variously merged together and fused into Tibetan Buddhism. Tibetan Buddhism, like all Buddhism is based on compassion for all sentient beings and contains many esoteric theories and practices of legendary mountain yogis.

Tibet and the surrounding region is a land of integration, where meditation practitioners spent most of their time in seclusion so as to develop their mind, body and spirit to the point of oneness, of fusion. These yogis and wise gurus are capable of amazing feats, including simply surviving in the extreme elevation Himalayan cold without heat or protection from the harsh mountainous elements. One of the first higher meditative practices in the esoteric Tibetan Buddhist yoga practice called Naropa yoga is the practice of inner fire, the creation of psychic heat, Tummo.

The Tummo meditation is exemplary of how much potential power individuation can lead to and is also exemplary of why institutions are occasionally frightened by such individual power. Though Tummo is effective in the Himalayas to make one basically impervious to cold, like many meditations, Buddhist and otherwise, its origins can be traced back to the hot climate of India. Martial arts, internal arts and Buddhism all originated in India, with roots beyond that possibly and were brought to Tibet, then China and the rest of Asia. Tummo was previously known as the warming breath of Khadomas in India.

In the distant past when learning tools were scarce, when even paper and pen were difficult to acquire, allegories and adages were implemented and passed from teacher to student as learning tools. Many of these adages were not so coincidentally of a teacher and student. Many now appear in Sufi parables and Zen koans. All of the adages are layered like onions, so that one can learn many things from the same concept over time as experience and comprehension expands. Today despite there being fewer teachers and fewer gurus there are more ways to learn and yet adages ultimately remain powerful learning tools layered with many lessons.

The following adage provides insight into how an adage can be more revelatory the more you comprehend. If ignorant of Tummo the adage is profound, but means only so much, when one comprehends Tummo it is revelatory of much more.

The student asks Master Tozan, "How can we escape from severe heat and severe cold?"

Master Tozan answers, "You have to go where there is no hot and no cold."

The student responds, "Where is the place where there is no hot or cold? Where is that true place of refuge for the mind?"

"When it is hot, become that heat completely! When it is cold, become one with that cold completely and totally! When it is painful, become that pain completely and totally, and when you are miserable, become that misery totally and completely! In the very midst of that, go beyond all the thoughts you hold in your mind, let go of all the ideas of good or bad or gain or loss – let go of all of these thoughts – and from there grasp that place of your very own vivid life energy! That which directly experiences pain, feel that life energy directly, grasp that life energy that feels that pain and sorrow."

Like all great adages and allegories revelatory of life and its predicaments it provides many lessons and insights, the major lesson revealing the importance of meditative acceptance for acceptance provides opportunity for integration. And with integration transmutation of weakness into strength is possible. All the meditative practices of 10,000 kicks within their core present the idea of transmutation of weakness into strength, similar to the alchemical idea of turning lead to gold. Only with acceptance can one escape from severe heat and cold through integration and transmutation, similar to the idea of taking lemons and fusing them with water and honey to make lemonade.

In every meditative practice, in every internal and external art there is first the development of self, then development of integration and then transmutation of weakness into strength. It is as if first one must hone oneself and gather the alchemical elements, the lead, the philosopher's stone and the fire, and then one can perform the transmutation into gold. First one must gather or practice for the transmutation.

Theory and practice and most importantly devotion to practice are required. For gathering balanced energy there are prerequisites. In chi gung theory it is said to take 100 days of devotional practice to first grow the figurative wheat and then integrate the harvest for initial transmutation into the bread, to grow the energy and then take advantage of it for sustenance. Some Tibetan yoga requires aspirants perform 108,000 full prostrations before moving forward in practice, 100,000 plus 8,000 to make up for mistakes and miscounting and to relate to 108, the most austere number. The devotion to prostrations and the repetition of meditative movements create chi, stimulate bioelectricity.

Taking on a practice of building energy is a serious business which one should not take too seriously. Devotion is tremendously important, but not everyone has 108,000 prostrations in them. A healing meditative movement is as simple as a prostration, the devotion being the most important aspect. Sometimes you need to heal yourself and such is very much like growing wheat, balancing everything may not work out perfectly, but more than likely you will benefit, maybe not as much as some, but surely you will have more to eat than those who did not attempt to grow at all or stopped half way through.

Naropa yoga is a series of esoteric Tibetan Buddhist meditations, practices and initiations organized into six forms or stages. Tummo is the first stage of Naropa yoga, metaphysical meditation practices during which the spiritual and physical planes are made to align for enlightenment. Naropa yoga makes up the primary methods used by some of the legendary wise yogis of mountain retreat who performed stupendous meditative acts of mind and body, such as going without food and water for long periods or mindreading or controlling the weather. Tummo is the scientifically validated practice of heat generation while in still meditation in a cold environment. Tummo is the first stage to imparting one's mindful will to overcome matter, in this case heat and cold.

The psychic heat of Tummo is followed by the yoga of the illusory body, the yoga of the dream state (this is comparable to lucid dreaming), yoga of the clear light, yoga of bardo (bardo is the stage between death and new birth) and yoga of the transference of consciousness. In each of the following meditations Tummo is utilized initially as a beginning meditation followed by whatever one of the other meditations the practitioner is absorbed in. Tummo enables complete control and complete integrative connection of mind, body, spirit and surroundings.

Tummo is practically necessary to learn in order to survive comfortably in the extreme Himalayan elements, but it is much more than controlling the physical generation of heat. Tummo yoga is the yoga of inner heat or the yoga of wisdom fire. Tummo enables the physical acceleration of heat generation, it allows one to literally overcome extreme cold, but it is just a beginning to psychic ability. I believe that Tummo helps to link the mind, body and spirit including of course the parasympathetic and sympathetic aspects of the nervous system allowing one to consciously control what was unconsciously controlled, such as regulation of body temperature. Tummo meditation quiets the chatter of the mind enabling one to be in the clear. This clarity instigates conscious control of former response mechanisms, in this case heat generation and instigates the beginning recognition of innate psychic abilities.

Tummo is accomplished essentially using the abstract of the Tozan adage; accept, clear everything, then perform transmutation. Tummo is explainable yet near impossible to do without extensive practice. Naropa yoga and all meditations are almost too complicated to communicate completely, one must experience them. Naropa yoga must be learned from a guru and practiced with devotion and minimal distraction. But anyone can feel Tummo's potential and many have. Remember when you first spoke in front of a large group or some other time where your temperature rose due to a lack of clarity in nervousness and imagine applying that power in clarity. Imagine that devotion to a meditation and meditative movement can lead to control of one's energy.

One of the normal guidelines for learning Naropa yoga is a three year retreat. The movements and mind state required in preparation to begin to attempt Tummo and the following aspects or stages of Naropa yoga are so complicated that direct instruction is normally the only way, normally, simply because the power of mindful consciousness can supersede anything including lacking instruction and lacking meditative isolation. The power of consciousness can create the strength to move a car, find psychic information in dreams without actively trying and create inner heat at will. And yet to harness our power usually requires practice, dedication and refinement. Today isolation of the mind in the mountains is nearly impossible, as is finding a proper guru.

Today it is difficult to learn meditative movement for developing the power of self and it is easy to be taught systems that steer us away from learning our true individual capacity. And because of this it is important to consider the quality of our teachers and what we are being taught relative to meditation and all things. However as it concerns meditative movement the quality of the students is a more important consideration than the quality of the teacher. A good teacher and a poor student leads to little progression, whereas a quality student learns many things from many people and in doing so, can often teach their teachers.

Isolation from distraction is important because we are weighed down by a complex arrangement of embedded conditioning and erratic stressors taught to us by society. Such distraction and bad teaching require meditation just to attain the open and clear state required before beginning to learn something like Tummo. Meditative movements bring us into the proper mind state to achieve quality consciousness so we can learn and so we can unlearn.

The Tibetan meditative movement of trul khor is traditionally a preparatory practice preceding Tummo and ngodro before it. Ngodro traditionally involves prostrations and meditations. Trul khor is a form of yoga, a series of primal meditative movements with some aspects similar to certain yoga and chi gung. The endeavors of learning Tummo or trul khor were never taken lightly. Vigorous and intense practice of precise internal and external positioning accompanied learning these practices beginning with Ngodro, consisting of meditations with direct lineage to Buddha.

Bodhicitta is a Tibetan Buddhist meditation passed down directly from Buddha. It is a basic meditation practice that is learned and integrated in later more complex meditations. Known as the seed of Buddha it is one of the best meditations in my experience and is reflected among many other differing practices. I was taught this meditation over a couple of days and I fear it is so profound I could never do it justice in my explanation, no matter how long, but it is so simple, so beautiful and so beneficial, I feel I have to at least include it here.

To begin, sit in cross legged position on a meditation pillow. Allow time to settle into absorption by relaxing and focusing on the breath. The rhythm of the following meditation consists of mindfulness of an idea followed by relaxing the mind, thinking on nothingness. The nothingness gives us a chance to relax, compared to thinking about the series of ideas ehich can all be quite intense. The flow of thought is like the Yin Yang symbolism of intensity and stillness. The process can be done in any time period. The point is to cover each idea as deeply as can be, given time or mental state circumstances.

The meditation is formed from important Buddhist concepts. Many meditations are derived from such teachings, Buddhist and otherwise, so that there are lessons in a sense for the secular, and meditative.

The first part of the meditation consists of concentration on each of The Four Thoughts; precious human body, impermanence, karma and samsara. This is done by focusing on the ideas through personal experiences and/or universal understandings. Every being is precious for spontaneous Buddhahood could happen, but humans are precious because we are capable of enlightenment; hence precious human body. After finding example of how we or others are precious, come to the point of gentle concentration on relaxation. Breathe in relaxed manner after the contemplation after contemplation on precious human body then proceed on to the impermanence idea, and then the pause again for gentle concentration on relaxation, and so on. Most people comprehend karma, however samsara is less widely known. Samsara is the plane of existence of suffering, of birth and death we are all in.

The second part of the meditation utilizes concentration on The Four Immeasurables in the same pattern of mindful focus followed by relaxation. There is a modification of the Four Immeasurables order of operation in the meditation, however. They are traditionally presented as; love for self, love for others, love for the happiness of others, and love for all beings in equanimity. In this meditation process begin by focusing on love for all beings in equanimity and end with love for self.

The third part of the meditation is Buddha breath. On every inhale imagine you are removing the ignorance and suffering of others, other people specifically, and those generally locally and globally. And on every exhale imagine you are sending them compassion and happiness. Imagine you are a conduit of Buddha or supreme consciousness. Imagine this is all done through you, instigated by you making the connection with above and below.

Imagine lotus flowers from Buddha consciousness being transported through you on every exhale and on every inhale the fiery pain and suffering is drawn into a fiery lotus flower that remains in front of you. This flower then burns up the ignorance and suffering drawn into it. Finish the meditation by keeping a lotus flower for yourself, and imagining light shining through you and onto you. Each step of the process can take as long as you like or as long as it takes to come to a realization through the first four concepts, send love through the second set of concepts and complete the Buddha Breathing that is inhaling suffering and exhaling healing as a seed of Buddha.

There are of course volumes written on the Four Thoughts and Four Immeasurables and I suggest seeking out more information on them if you decide to delve into this simple and profound meditation, directly passed down from Buddha. These concepts are some of the most simple and most profoundly deep. After this meditation and others I like to imagine washing off my being of any excess ignorant suffering that might have stuck to me, with light.

In Lama Anagarika Govinda's book The Way of The White clouds he describes a monk as saying that beginning a practice of devotion like meditation, meditative movement and compassionate existence is essentially like becoming a snake and winding one's way through a tube which leads in two directions. In one direction is bliss and in the other direction is hell. This is accompanied by, from my experience, the occasional feeling of discomfort in being so confined in a tube no matter which way you're going. Proceeding down a path of self-development can be at times uncomfortable and restrictive like a tube.

The fact that beginning a practice of dedication is like a tube stems from the fact that life is like a tube, in many ways. We are already born into an allegorical tube, only most are not sensitive enough to realize it and most don't want to address it. We are already in the tube like predicament of mortality, destined for bliss or suffering. This snakelike spiritual positioning of practice is akin to our physical positioning in life. We are born as a snake in a mortality tube.

Practicing meditative movement brings awareness in total, including awareness of mortality. Initially this can be uncomfortable, but this is only temporary. Heightened awareness is like getting a deep massage. We may think we are experiencing vitality, but when we get a massage we realize how tight and constricted we are and then are loosened and relieved. Initially metaphysically linking the mind, body and spirit can result in discomfort from heightened awareness in the same way a deep massage initially results in unease and ultimately healing. Heightened awareness is at first frightening, but leads to bliss. In Buddhism awareness of death is part of the greatest lessons and leads to compassionate being while the opportunity is here.

Metaphorically speaking our energy is often compared to a snake for snakelike energy is said to spiral up and down us. The symbolism of rising and twisting kundalini energy from our grounded root chakra spiraling upwards and the caduceus symbol of winged snakes representing healing still used in modern medicine are familiar examples. We are all like snakes in a tube, knowing our position allows comfort as we go.

Massive preparation is normally undertaken for Tummo, massive activation of the meditative mind state, enhancement of consciousness and quieting of mind chatter. This is done not necessarily because one begins as incapable before practice, but because it is believed such energetic practices, though simple physically and not entirely complex mentally, build up and release energy in powerful metaphysical ways and in the same way karma. This build up, similar to ischemic pressure in massage can be dangerous if you're unprepared for such an intense release. Meditative movement develops coordination between in hand and feet movement, such coordination and devotion opens up the meridians, our ability to handle energy.

The meditative movements in Tibetan Fusion are totally simple and primal, requiring only that you are capable of doing them. They can be integrated in preparation for powerful meditation such as Tummo or utilized to prepare one for whatever in life as they are all like common denominators. Tummo is highly complex and demonstrative of our psychic powers. I feel I learn things best when revealed complex matters first, just as food for thought and as a possible goal, then begin to learn the theory and practice of what I am prepared for. Consider Tummo as a goal for some that one can be aware of and Tibetan Fusion as an integrative practice anyone can do and variously benefit from.

Tummo and such powerful practices have interested and frightened individuals for generations. Powerful individuals can disturb others who seek power and those who fear it. Wherever there were battles secrets arose so as to gain advantage. Such interaction is part of the reason there are so many secrets among the internal and martial arts, why teaching is often limited and perhaps, at least in part, why many practitioners retreat to mountain isolation. Sometimes information is withheld because readiness is questioned, most frequently though information is withheld because of reactions by dastardly individuals and institutions. Today however, in the battle we all fight, as individuals among institutions, information must be shared.

Tummo meditation is not recommended for just anyone, not because it is a secret so much anymore, but because it takes preparation and requires precaution to move energy. A quality mental and physical state is required for Tummo, just as you learn to swim in calm waters before going into the ocean and attempting to surf. A mind body connection through prior meditative practices is absolutely necessary to learn how to surf the ocean break and perform Tummo. Tummo, Naropa yoga, trul khor, and practically all forms of meditative movement are very much like surfing the ocean break, it can be graceful or terrible.

All meditative movements have all had secret aspects to their practice which began as ways to preserve them, but often ended up resulting in distortion or near elimination. Sometimes the information was held by close knit circles for the powers could be misused and sometimes the authorities of the day forced the practice itself to go underground. Today the cultural war on Tibet has released the practices to the world which were once held in secret. Though distortion and misunderstanding is possible, such is better than elimination, and such is potentially no worse than the distortion and misunderstandings sometimes resulting from keeping secrets. Many great teachers, gurus and lamas, who were once only allowed to teach a select few, are being released from this karmic bond and being allowed to reveal Tibetan meditative movements to the world so that the authorities of China cannot destroy the practices altogether.

Tummo is complex, but some of it, physically speaking, is totally basic. In order to attempt Tummo learn and practice tai chi, chi gung, trul khor or kung fu and/or yoga. In order to attempt Tummo you have to be in a heightened energetic state. After learning and practicing meditative movement in coordination with the breath, multiple forms of meditation and gaining some hint of control over the sympathetic and parasympathetic systems one might be ready to begin to at least experience Tummo and build some imperviousness to cold. Tummo is serious business, but one experiences it just as a child experiences a fun game, with a smile.

In chi gung there is a practice called snowbathing which builds one's ability to maintain body heat. Snowbathing is one prerequisite to Tummo and can be done to enhance the practice. Simply immerse oneself or relax in the snow wearing nothing but bathing suit. Do so laughing with the anticipation of being involved in a game, then try to warm yourself through meditative movement and conscious mind state in a relatively cool environment. After snowbathing a few times, eventually try to warm yourself without movement, only meditation. One can imagine the physical exertion required for this practice and I do not recommend it just want to share knowledge of it.

To experience Tummo or build imperviousness to cold bathe in cold water, take a snowbath or expose yourself to cold environment however possible and then sit in a simple meditative position in temperatures around 60 degrees Fahrenheit as opposed to temperatures approaching freezing. In the beginning it is best to perform some kind of meditative movement, not necessarily anything vigorous, but something to enhance movement of subtle energy. Wear dry normal clothing or just a dry sheet. Sit cross legged or in a full lotus, or whatever variation of cross legged you're most comfortable in. Sit on a cushion or folded blanket for comfort.

Place your hands on top of your thighs with the backside of your wrists pressing on your inner thigh with the pointer finger extended inward so as to straighten your back and open the energy channels. Remain in this position for several breaths while pressing downward. Bring your hands cupped together at your belly or root chakra, right palm on top for men, left on top for women or set your palms to your knees.

After slowing down the breath and achieving a relaxed state begin to meditate on being totally hollow. Physically we are not totally hollow, but spiritually we can be totally hollow or as in the Tozan adage, 'let go of all thoughts and clear ourselves.' The powerful meditative understanding demonstrated in Tummo and suggested in many other practices is clearing all emotions and all thoughts to the point of being hollow, completely clear. On being clear of all the emotions and thoughts, clear on the spiritual plane, one can harness the energy it took to create and deal with the emotions and thoughts that the clarity and transform that energy into the inner fire of Tummo, for even just a portion of the energy required for feeling and thinking is enough to create the inner fire when applied correctly to clarity.

The potential power of our inner emotions and thoughts to make heat is recognizable in recalling the time you first had to be an orator or were nervous for other reasons and started sweating. And it can be most notable in the moment you felt lonely after you were newly made single and saw your ex with their new love interest. Such intense moments illustrate the power we can manifest. Clearing all emotions and thoughts unshackles burdens preventing us from being in control.

Once you can visualize hollowness and clarity imagine all the energy it took to fill the mind with thoughts and emotional distractions, good and bad, and imagine that energy being transformed into a single spark and a very small, very powerful flame. Imagine the spark sized fire within you grows in intensity and fills one with heat as any fire in any enclosed and hollow space would. Imagine the spark of fire comes to and originates from the middle of your being, your heart chakra. Further imagine there are three vertical lines of energy running up and down along your spine. Imagine these channels of flowing energy begin to glow and emit heat as well. The channels extend from the base of your tailbone to the crown of your head and intersect through each of your main chakras. Imagine they are the width of a single strand of your hair, then your finger, then your arm, then imagine them taking up your entirety and then setting fire to the entirety of one's external surroundings, then imagine the sea of fire returning into you filling you, then coming into the coils of an arm's width, then your finger, your hair and one single point.

You can flex your body to initiate some stimulation if you feel like it, remaining in the same position, just bringing alternating tension and relaxation to your muscles. Initially try to slow and regulate the breath so that inner clarity and relaxation is possible. Bring the thoughts and breath together as one by thinking, 'I am breathing in, I am breathing out. I am taking a long/short breath in/out. I am inhaling with all. I am exhaling with all,' or similar sentiments in a relaxed and aware state.

When you have lengthened and steadied the breath for clarity you can begin to expand your exhalations so they are twice as long as your inhalations. While doing this also practice Taoist reverse breathing, expanding the diaphragm on exhalation and contracting inwardly on the inhalation. After breathing in that cycle for a time, you can intermittently incorporate bellows breathing; short, quick inhalations and exhalations, so quickly that you complete three breath cycles per second. Practice bellows breathing for fifteen seconds initially and longer when and if it is comfortable. Bellows breathing is extremely powerful, take care and begin slowly with it.

After completing bellows breathing return to Taoist reverse breathing cycle and then incorporate a lengthy pause on reaching lung capacity. Hold your breath, at 85% capacity and breath out as slowly as possible. Normal breathing should be conducted from about 0% to about 85% capacity. Throughout Tummo one should retain a small percentage of breath locked in the diaphragm and let it be like retention of fuel for the flame. After conducting this breathing pattern for a time including intermittent bellows breathing, change the pattern so that the intermittent bellows breathing punctuates slow deep breathing that includes a pause in the middle of the inhalation, keeping the same timing of exhalations being twice as long as inhalations.

The ancients measured breath in heartbeats. One form of chi gung (chi gung means life force cultivation) breathing describes increasing one's breath cycle, including pauses, to 100 heartbeats per breath for extended life and rejuvenation further reaching for 1000 heartbeats per breath cycle is said to be the goal to reach near immortality.

Imagine the breath as fueling the flame and eventually as integrated with flame itself. Imagine the breath with pause on full inhalation relates to a microcosmic orbit and that the pause dividing the inhalation into two parts relates to a macrocosmic orbit. If it suits you imagine the lower three chakras are circulating and radiating incredible heat with the micro and that the four other major chakras circulate and radiate immense and intense heat into the macrocosmic circulation.

Early Tibetan ideas noted four base chakras, most energy concepts today point to seven base chakras. The four chakras correlate with the crown (crown and third eye are often mutual in Tibetan tradition), throat, heart and sacrum chakras among the more commonly known basic seven. These chakras are likened to wheels of a chariot as well as to the four elements earth, wind, fire and water. It is said that one can stimulate Tummo by concentrating on opening these chakras like an umbrella and spinning them, clockwise, like chariot wheels. It's said that their alchemical unification assists enlightenment and heat generation.

It is interesting to contemplate too that the chakras wheels, no matter how many are noted, are aligned one on top of the other Later, spinning in a stacked manner rather than spinning like interwoven clockwork. There is also a five chakra System widely theorized among Tibetan Buddhists. The five chakra system includes the concept of the root chakra.

Perhaps the Five Tibetan Rites are meant to correlate with the concept of activating five chakra system to optimum spin.

The other energy points were not unconsidered in total just unconsidered as primary. You can consider the four chakras as the primary of the seven which in turn are the primary points among thousands all over the body. Each of these four, seven and thousands of energy points or chakras can generate heat. If one is unfamiliar with chakras or have more of an analytical mind conceptualize that each of the trillions of individual cells which make up your physical are capable of generating heat –at your metaphysical command. Another powerful visualization in accordance with the ideas in Tummo or at least in beginning training towards Tummo, is based on the understanding that we all originate as stardust, we all are composed of elements which have undergone a process of development and decay billions of years in the making, a transformation of stars into conscious living beings. Remember we are all made up of stardust; visualize the heat giving potential of stars within you.

Imagine a connection with the universal macrocosm, the fire from the sun and stars radiating through you, through the crown of your head. Imagine everything directly around you is on fire because your skin is glowing hot. Imagine the heat is so intense and your body (physical/spiritual) is so clear that the flame and heat transpose physical/spiritual borders. Imagine that the heat being generated and absorbed by the chakras is so intense they literally alight and burn up completely clearing all blockages within every layer of each chakra. This obtains further clarity for the burned chakras are immediately replaced by newly clarified points of energy infused with universal sun energy. The Tummo practice empowers individuals to the point that outside influences, including extreme cold, do not alter the individual's state of being. It enables complete body control and allows one to live comfortably in the Himalayan cold and most importantly enhances the physical/spiritual connection leading to further psychic ability. Tummo enables control of physical mechanisms which normally run automatically and the mind which normally runs endlessly.

Tibetan Fusion is not trul khor or Naropa yoga. It is not even a hybridization of such secretive Tibetan instructions though that label is acceptable if labels are required. It is however a culmination of many practices, a confluence of practices and forms to allow open access to energy. Tibetan Fusion is a key to open up your energy flows and at the very least bring about renewed physical vitality along with relaxation. Tibetan Fusion is designed for the newcomer to meditation and mind body connection and yet long time practitioners of body movement and/or meditation can also benefit from Tibetan Fusion for it is a combination of primal movements which are easily integrated into your current practice. Tibetan Fusion is designed for those who find themselves hampered by the burden of age, limited by time restraints or a physical deterioration or injury and yet it can be beneficial to Olympic level athletes as well.

From the confluence of Tibet, Northern India and Southern China come some of the most powerful and inspirational meditative practices and not so coincidently come some of the most magical tales of superhuman capabilities, of psychic recognition, miraculous healing and seemingly impossible physical feats. And yet the ancient practices of tai chi, chi gung and yoga all suggest that such potential is a simple matter of refinement of the individual.

Tantric philosophy opens and undoes limits whether through yoga or other learning. Tantra means implies union and fusion; acceptance, integration and transmutation. When one is able to freely accept and integrate learning one is bettered for it. The more rigidly one chooses information the more limited one becomes, the more incapable one is of learning and the more incapable one is in general. This principle can be applied to philosophy, or meditative movement, or love, or life. And in this way tantra is one of the most powerful systems as well as one of the oldest philosophies, being open to fusion.

Many of the most basic meditative movements have already been integrated among many meditative practices with occasionally slight modifications. Simple movements do not limit, but allow easy and open access to energy. Simplicity doesn't mean you gain access to a different place, simplicity means you gain access to the same building in a less complicated manner. Integration of simple movements with unified principles enhances one's potential energy access, simplicity allows for easy integration, not limitation. The primary meaning of the word yoga is union, suggestive of integration of the body and mind, the physical with the spiritual. The more meditative movements and history of one learns one realizes that they all originated from a few sources and most were integrated and expanded on, like languages. The more one practices one realizes that the energy comes in many forms or qualities, but it is the same energy.

Integration of simplicity is powerful and beneficial. Simple integrative approaches to diet work the best for health and longevity. It is best to eat many different types of simple foods prepared simply. There are a few foods which are best eaten by themselves, but we all need a wide variety of foods and function best when we have access to such. The combination of many simple foods throughout the day is the best way to obtain nutrition.

When slightly or moderately sickened, probably at least in part due to a lack of variety in diet, we chop, dice, blend, heat and fuse numerous simple ingredients into a soup because it's healing. The same theory for diet is applicable to meditative movements. The combination of simple ingredients into a soup can provide easy access to the required nutrients to heal and a combination of simple meditative movements can help to easily assimilate healing energy the same. Neither the nutrients in the soup or energy in movements are deficient due to integration.

Many meditative movements might appear too complex to attract as many people as they should or could. The time and commitment involved to learn and integrate the movements as one's own keys to opening doors can sometimes appear as too hefty a burden. Most people are seeking to lessen their burden, so as soon as they can convince themselves that such practices are burdensome, they will turn away from them as superfluous and time consuming. Such practices however lend to a happier and enhanced mind state resulting in enhanced wellbeing. Meditative movements initially take time, but immediately make you feel better when doing other things. Meditative movements at first seem to take time, but in reality make time, they supply you with more focus so you accomplish things easier and quicker and they supply you with more energy so you sleep better and require less sleep.

Bruce Lee designed Jeet Kune Do, a fighting style combining and refining many styles of martial arts. It is an integration and transmutation, a river formed from many creeks, streams and confluences. He took his knowledge of martial arts combined with new and powerful correlative ideas and then refined, and fused together to form a more practical and powerful system.

Tibetan Fusion is an energy building practice combining elementary aspects of chi gung, tai chi and yoga. Tibetan Fusion is similar to what Bruce Lee accomplished in martial arts with Jeet Kune Do, only Tibetan Fusion is a combination of healing arts rather than a martial art. Instead of combining self-defense practices I have combined self-healing practices and meditation understandings and boiled them down to be the most palatable for the Western mind, the easily distracted, ego driven, hyper busy over-thinker.

Tibet has always been a land of integration and fusion, the roof of the world, the peak of spirituality. Tibetan culture was sculpted from the primordial shamanism of the Bonn religion combined with the compassionate wisdom of Buddhism. Think of Tibetan Fusion and all meditative movement as akin to this Tibetan combination. Think of being a natural and primordial Earth being with complete universal compassionate consciousness. No matter how the world has changed and how we have changed it, our bodies, our consciousness machines, are the same biological design ancient meditative movements were originally conceived for. And the highest mind state to have is still compassion. Compassion results in bettered state of being and open compassion also results in fearlessness, a feeling which alone builds energy.

In Tibetan Buddhism the flaming sword is symbolic for cutting through shields and encasements of ignorance as opposed to through armor and flesh, ignorance based on superfluous assumptions. A warrior approaches the state of fearlessness by raising their sword, however true fearlessness resides in compassion, in removing ignorance and hatred, the most frequent origins of fear, making the physical sword into a spiritual or metaphysical sword. Practice meditative movement with the mind state of a compassionate warrior towards being open in fearless, equal compassion and you will likely be rewarded.

Tibetan culture represents the best of the world, a totally peaceful state based on spirituality, based on believing that every life is precious and we will likely come back here and reincarnate when we die. So instead of living to complete bucket lists and polluting totality as if it doesn't matter, without consideration for the future, Tibetans care for all in compassion. But Tibet has been culturally raided and globalized, just like the rest of the world. All indigenous cultures for the last six hundred years or so have been pacified and homogenized and often eliminated in genocidal terms that to mention them all would be a task of impossibility for so many have been wiped out entirely leaving barely a trace.

Tibet is an indigenous and compassionate nation being effectively streamlined and forced to walk in line with the rest of us and if not for the political and geological landscape it might have been so sooner. Tibet was a nation based on compassion and spirituality. Tibet was a nation of people who lived in the harshest environment in near total cooperation with one system, that of spirituality. About 1 in 6 Tibetans sought to be monks and study in one of the thousands of mountain monasteries, many of which were destroyed. So many people were able to walk the spiritual path because the whole of society believed that reaching for such devoted ascension was the pinnacle of being and contributed to the process assisting the pursuits.

Tibet is a nation of fusion at the crossroads of Asia with China to the north and India to the south, both places of diversity on their own. But today, like the nations of Afghanistan and Palestine in particular it is a land undergoing assimilation, takeover and gentrification instead of fusion and oneness. Because many of the Tibetan Buddhists, yogis, gurus and lamas either ran away or were killed and because their isolation for meditation was disturbed, because they were not allowed to teach the next generation and because the Tibetan culture is being lawfully disintegrated information on Tibetan practices are being shared with the impetus to reveal the practices so they are not disappeared. The karmic bonds which prevented masters from teaching just anyone have been released. With this in mind and considering the knowledge we have on other meditative movements, never before in history has so much knowledge been available on meditation and assimilation.

In sharing information comes the possibility of all out adulteration of what was mostly pure. However in sharing information the practices cannot be destroyed. There is also the possibility that sharing information on meditative movement leads to greater understanding of energy entirely and allows access for some that would otherwise not know about it or seek it.

One's specific practice is important and yet the devotion to practice with a positive mind state is perhaps more of a key component to development. The movements are indeed often secondary to devotion. Meditative movements must activate certain Humanity is a fusion. What we call pure and centric is often from somewhere else and has been long ago mixed up. The Tibetan Fusion program is designed to help the Western mind develop a practice to build their energy simply, but there are 10,000 sets of 10,000 kicks.

There is the story of a wise man who on reaching a certain point of mastery and devotion was required to travel and reach out to people outside his area. This is one variation: one day after traveling for a time he reached a great lake and heard of hermit who was on an island in the middle of it. The hermit was said to be an aesthetic devoting his time to meditation. The wise man decided to take a boat to see the hermit. On meeting the wise man the hermit was very excited and asked many questions. The wise man and hermit had a lengthy conversation consisting primarily of the hermit inquiring of the wise man. The two eventually meditated together at which time the hermit realized he had been reciting a certain mantra the wrong way. The wise man corrected the hermit and soon after he departed. The wise man returned to the awaiting boat and set forth on the water. Feeling satisfied the wise man spoke with the boatman and enjoyed the lake's beauty. They were in the middle of the lake when the wise man noticed the boat man stop in awe. The hermit approached them, "Wait!" he exclaimed running up to the boat, walking on water, "How does the correct mantra go again?"

The point is that proper pronunciation does not lead to walking on water, it is proper devotion. The actual devotional practice, the specific pronunciation, is often less important than how devoted you are. The pronunciation of the mantra and the perfection of body movement are much less important than being devoted to the process and practicing with a compassionate mind state.

Tibetan Fusion isn't true Tibetan Yoga, in fact the Five Tibetan Rites of Rejuvenation, a part of Tibetan Fusion may not even be of Tibetan origin. The series of movements may be from another neighboring culture of Tibet, Nepal or Bengal perhaps. And the series now has a sixth posture, a movement known as a bandha in yoga, as opposed to a breath coordinated positioning or asana. A yoga asana is a body position. Bandhas are movements or body mechanical switches of internal energy. The origin of most meditative movements is often unknown with known integrations and additions. The origins however are less important compared with their ability to instill balanced energy. The Five Rites of Rejuvenation despite their mysterious origins have notable benefits.

Tibetan Fusion is a series of simple practices, a fusion of chi gung, tai chi, the Five Tibetan Rites, various yoga and other primal practices which instill devotion and build energy. Tibetan Fusion is one of many paths to the top of the mountain, one which is suitable as well as soothing to the often rushed and frantic mind state of today. Tibetan yoga, Yantra yoga and Naropa yoga and all meditative movements are highly developed systems which are all valuable for the development of individuals and humanity as a whole. And mainly so because of the meditation, the meditation you make your own.

The lesson of integration of is sharing and openness to the oneness. And it's a powerful lesson for all humanity. We need to share information and materials more, and accept each other more. We need to clear the thoughts and emotions which form blockages and accept each another. If we do not share and accept we will have nothing. Integration is accepting and sharing. The cultural revolution of China inspired homogenization and even elimination of indigenous culture including that of Tibet, not integration, not acceptance or sharing. The institutions of the Western world typically operated in the same way, not to necessarily single out China.

For thousands of years practitioners of tai chi, chi gung and yoga have only been able to bestow their information to a few people at a time. For thousands of years the teachings all came with warnings that if done improperly there could be dire consequences. And this is true, but what they fail to mention is that not doing them at all can be much worse. What is often unmentioned is that we will all find ourselves as the proverbial snake in the tube eventually. Buddhism or Buddhist meditations are often part of prerequisite for aspiring yoginis before learning Tummo or what have you. Part of the reason for this, I believe from my experience only, is that these Buddhist meditations present a step by step process for compassion. And in order to be open to energy, to hold it and offer it, one must be open to all things. Open compassion allows one to be open to energy.

No master begins as such. It is refined repetition which makes the master masterful. Hardly any master invents independently, but all masters can mimic. Mimicry is how many postures and movements were initially conceptualized, mimicry of the elements, animals and mimicry of our true nature. We are such profound mimickers we even mimic negative behavior and do so without realization.

Tibetan Fusion is a combination of simple meditative movements. Each ingredient is on its own benevolent. And each is easy to learn, mimic and adopt as yours. The ingredients are not meals onto themselves, the combination of which could cause gastrointestinal discomfort. The ingredients are leaves, stems, roots and fruits from different plants grown in the same garden.

There are certain dynamics which one should follow and principles one should understand, but in learning, the most important thing to do is to begin just as the most important thing to do when you need sustenance is to eat. The benefits from practicing meditative movements are many and beyond simply physical. Many times one will not notice the benefits or mistake them for something else. But eventually through practice you will reap undeniable rewards. Refinement and repetition makes what was first difficult to remember and perform second nature, then more and more subtleties and connections can be made. Beginning a practice is in an inspiration to learn and become your own master of your own meditation.

"People's natures are basically the same, it is their practices which sets them far apart."
~Confucius

Meditation and Breath

The easiest thing for most people to do is watch television. Television takes the emotions and thoughts away to distant sitcoms, away from the here and now while we sit calm. When you are in a meditative mind state watching television is one of the most difficult things to do. It operates by distraction, by removing us from the present and taking us to mostly upsetting and/or dramatic situations.

In taking us away watching television generally makes one of the most difficult things for most people to do, more difficult; being present in meditation. Meditation brings us into the present, television takes us away from our presence. Meditation becomes difficult because of how distant and distracted we are from constant mediation of television and increasingly frantic life experience. Watching television takes us away from ourselves to a fantasy, away from reality. Television and all mediation make it more difficult to be ourselves. We become immersed in the program directly and momentarily and held by the programming over the long term.

Watching television is one of many things a busy mind will do so as not to have to face itself and its shadows. Mediation of television takes us away, it removes our individual power and our individualism, but makes it so we do not have to face ourselves, which for many is a fair enough trade off. And the longer we go watching television, the longer we live in distraction without facing our shadows, the bigger the shadows become and harder to face they seem. Meditation is one of the easiest, most pleasing and most empowering activities, enabling our true individual potential. Meditation is energizing and relaxing at the same time, watching television primarily dulls energy and limits relaxation, the extreme of which can be noted in such programming invading your dreams. Meditation balances and brings us closer to ourselves. Television, mediation and life's distractions do the exact opposite.

Meditation is as easy as walking and as consciousness vehicles it's a process we were possibly biologically designed for, perhaps as much as we were meant to walk. Meditation is easy, but there are stages of meditation which require and lead to facing inward aspects of ourselves, facing our shadows, which can be just about the most difficult processes one can undergo. The process of shedding layers of ignorance is as difficult and rewarding as a snake shedding its skin. The traumas of life and distractions of living, often in as little as watching television, cocoon us in layers of ignorance, clouding the mind. Clearing such is difficult, but only part of the learning process, like stumbling.

Meditation metaphysically links our wandering thoughts and emotions with our physical in the natural here and now. As you meditate try to be present and remember that the physical is always here and now, it is our thoughts and feelings that wander. In meditation the idea is to calm the mind and activate consciousness. Meditation is a process and at first simply quieting the mind so to then peer inward can take a long time.

Meditation is easy or as easy to learn as walking. Being mentally and emotionally present can be difficult partly due to the influx of distracting experiences reducing our meditative mind state and potential relaxation. Meditation is easy, but one of the initial components of facing oneself can be a truly tumultuous procedure, the longer one has been distracted from self, the more difficult it potentially may be to face oneself. In learning to walk stumbling occurs, but no one gives up learning to walk, we simply learn what falling is like too. The following quotes are helpful to gently think on as one faces shadows and feels a sense of stumbling during meditation and in general.

"This too will pass." ~Buddha

"The affairs of the world will go on forever. Do not delay the practice of meditation." ~Milarepa

"When one comes to think of it, one cannot help feeling that nearly half the misery of the world would disappear if we, fretting mortals, knew the virtue of silence. Before modern civilization came upon us, at least six to eight hours of silence out of twenty four were vouchsafed to us. Modern civilization has taught us to convert night into day and golden silence into brazen din and noise. What a great thing it would be if we in our busy lives, could retire into ourselves for at least a couple of hours, and prepare our minds to listen to the voice of the great silence. The divine radio is always singing if we could only make ourselves ready to listen to it, but it is impossible to listen without silence." ~Gandhi

"As long as there is saliva in your mouth, it is never too late." ~Chinese Parable

"Perceiving brings one to the goal." ~Confucius

Within all moving or still meditation, there is mental movement, beginning with imagination, a shift into a mental state of being that one cannot see physically. There is also physical movement that is mostly invisible to the naked eye involving shifting and locking internal organ and glandular pressure variously. The Tummo meditation requires all sorts of preparation and activity, much of it invisible, but a quiet and open mind is the main goal of such. A quiet and open mind allows access to consciousness where the real potential power resides. Imagination always precludes action. In Tummo and meditation imagination is important. However everything from your home to yourself, were all firstly imagination before fruition. Moving chi or life energy happens in the same manner. Accessing the power of consciousness requires dedicated cultivation of imagination and action.

Meditation and meditative movement are performed to access the power of consciousness, to quiet the mind, but there are many roads and rivers to cross before reaching your true power. Before one can access your true potential, to the point one's focus cannot be unraveled, consider spending just about as much time in meditation as one has spent watching television so as to counter the mediations and distractions of programming.

Because of our physical predicament, requiring sustenance and satisfaction, ever subject to distraction and desire, meditative monks seek retreat to develop their energetic and spiritual potential, retreat for meditation to quiet the mind so as to access the power of consciousness. Our consciousness is a microcosmic reflection of the unfathomable and boundless universe. Being alone and quiet, away from the worldly ways of mediation and distraction is optimal to build connection with the unlimited boundlessness of consciousness.

Harnessing the power can be incredibly difficult requiring mental, physical and spiritual development of which isolation from negativity and negative distractions is extremely important. Much of life can be distracting and upsetting which is why meditation practitioners go on isolated retreats to monasteries of sorts or caves or take vows of silence or just seek a quiet place to meditate undisturbed for a moment. Isolation in meditation brings us inward where the real power resides, the real insights and real inspiration.

The access to the power of consciousness is nearly always clouded by desires and traumas held by the mind. Liberation is experienced by burning through the cloudiness like sunshine. Before we are able to access the boundlessness power within we are convinced that true power is outside ourselves through most mediation. We tend to lose parts of our potential power in life, often early in life. When we practice meditation feelings of youthful exuberance, curiosity and equal compassion for all existence return, because parts lost or distant return.

The worldly ways of institutionalization removes our individualism and replaces it with materialism. We yield our power to outside institutions instead of building on it inside ourselves. This predicament is nothing new. All adepts of absorption, (alternative understanding of meditation) all artists, scientists, philosophers and likely every Saint there ever was have all sought and advised one seek isolation from the worldly ways of the majority, many specifically recommending to avoid cities altogether. Potentially the oldest documented person to have ever lived, Li Ching Yun, advised people to avoid cities and worldly ways as it would shorten one's years and surely if alive today he would add television the list of things to avoid.

Most people fear isolation and dread loneliness, part of the reason television is constantly on for many. Most people are also surrounded by negative emotions/thoughts and desires of their own and others. And most people do all they can to avoid thinking about this, filling every moment with unthinking activity or simply the distraction of television. If you ever have practiced performing an athletic feat requiring one be present and focused you realize how easily we can distract ourselves or be distracted by others in a flicker of a moment. Remaining focused is sometimes the only thing that separates a homerun from a strikeout. And meditation enables such present focus.

Being isolated should not be feared. Yet being alone with negative emotions/thoughts and desires without anyone and without television to displace them is frightening. Isolation offers simple and efficient opportunity for reflection and introspection. Complexity brings further distraction to the fact of negativity, whereas isolation allows us time to face the shadows of ourselves. Without facing one's shadows one cannot be clear and without clearing through meditative isolation the burden of institutionalization, mediation or outright trauma might never be removed and developing inner power might not be possible. Facing the shadows of ourselves can be an upsetting endeavor often without any immediately quantifiable results. The first step in meditation is to realize the power within and the hindrances that need clearance. Isolation, even in moments of absorption, allows us to face negativity and in doing so begin to accept, integrate and transmute so as to be liberated.

Be positive when you meditate in a quiet isolated place. Be so positive that if there is occasional traffic where you are the noise just goes by. And just the same be so positive that as thoughts come up, let them go by like traffic or like waves then absorbed into the ocean. Be centered and focused.

"The ego is a monkey catapulting through the jungle. Totally fascinated by the realm of the senses, it swings from one desire to the next, one conflict to the next, one self-centered idea to the next. If you threaten it, it actually fears for its life. Let this monkey go. Let the senses go. Let desires go. Let conflicts go. Let ideas go. Let the fiction of life and death go. Just remain in the center, watching. And then forget that you are there." ~Lao Tzu

Realize the power within you as a literal conductor of electrical chi. Be present. Relax the mind and body, try to calm the fluttering thoughts and clear the stressed blockages. Imagine you are grounded to the earth and connected through a line or cord to the sun or your own star as a conduit of energy. Be relaxed and energized as you are rooted to the Earth and connected to the light at the same time.

The tai chi principle of relaxation teaches to calmly be aware of your overall positioning as you conduct meditative movement and throughout your daily activities. The tai chi principle of relaxation describes the mindset and body-set of being on point or being balanced. Mastery of an activity results in effortless performance. This effortless perfection is what is meant by relaxation in tai chi.

Relaxation and effortless performance results from balance. As with any activity, sport or otherwise, one has to strike a balance between form and function or method and style. Imagine this as a horizontal line with 'form' on one end and 'function' on the other end. One also has to develop a balanced approach to the matter, via managing tense and limp positioning. Imagine this as vertical line with tense at the top end and limp at the bottom. Now imagine the lines intersect and the optimal point of being is that point in the middle of each, the point of intersection. Balancing the horizontal line of form and function and the vertical line of tense and limp is relaxation. Watching television is not relaxation, it is mediation.

A similar cross reference model can be used to maintain a relaxed heart and mind state. Imagine that your individual consciousness is vertical while the consciousness of others, whether mass consciousness of a great collective, or small group or one other individual relates with our individual consciousness horizontally. If you are rooted vertically and in the sun then imbalanced or upsetting outside influences with be less likely to throw you off and distract you. The higher our vibration, the more rooted we are and more access to light we have, the less likely outside influences will shake us.

There are countless specific forms of meditation done moving and still, however there are just four basic physical positions for meditation; sitting, lying, standing, and walking. Sitting cross legged is one of the most common positions for meditation, try doing so on a cushion set on the floor at first. You can also sit on a chair with your hands on your knees. Try meditating lying flat on your back palms up fingertips touching the ground. A typical standing meditation can be done with your feet shoulder width apart, knees slightly bent, with your arms down fingertips touching fingertips at your navel. Walking meditation, as any meditative movement is more elaborate. Trying gently holding your elbows with your fingertips, arms crossed just in front of you and walk as softly and slowly as possible with a slight twist from the navel initiating each step. Be attentive to every micro movement try to make it so each step mimics the other equally.

There are four basic mental positions for meditation too. Frequently meditation is about clearing through the mind, through the thoughts and feelings, to connect with oneself and be present. Other times it is about finding something outside oneself, perhaps a solution to a problem. The four mental positions of meditation are formed via the intersection of these two types of applications of mindfulness and focus. The first application is one of mental fullness or mental emptiness. Meditation with mental fullness crowds the mind with an idea. Meditation with mental emptiness clears the mind of all ideas. The second application is of inward and outward concentration. One peers inward or outward with either a clear or crowded mind. Most meditation promotes a clear mind while peering inward. Certain forms of Sufi meditation crowd the mind peering outward. One way to solve problems is in this way, imagining the dilemma and a solution. Albert Einstein famously would perform thought experiments crowding his mind with ideas and imagining experiments. Psychic meditation clears the mind while peering outward. Healing meditation practices crowd the mind with an image of healing while peering inward for self and outwardly for others.

There are numerous forms of meditation, each efficient at problem solving in the world and potentiating our development or solving problems within to one degree or another. Yet whatever the specific variation of meditation is practiced one either crowds the mind or clears the mind, while peering inward or outward. And no matter what meditation you learn and practice, remember your own meditation, in line with certain guidelines, is the most powerful form for you. Relaxed awareness of the four physical positions and four mental positions of mediation can hone and enhance one's practices. The knowledge can also raise meditative mindfulness and conscious intent when you're not actively meditating, in life.

Relaxed awareness is essential in all forms of meditation, whether Einstein thought experiments or Zen stillness, whether for external problem solving or internal insight or healing. Awareness of the four forms of one's physical and mental positioning enhances meditation. Without physical focus and mental intention one will end up going in the wrong direction or walking in circles. Perhaps even more important than knowing your physical and mental positioning according to well established traditions, is the calm awareness of your breath. The first rule of still meditation is to practically always breathe through your nose. And generally one should keep your mouth shut and tongue on the roof of your mouth without tension in your mouth or jaw.

In yoga, tai chi and chi gung breath is explored in physical terms as well as spiritual terms. People tend to breathe in one of four ways. There is high breathing or collarbone breathing. This expends the most energy and obtains the least oxygen. Secondly there is mid breathing or rib breathing. It is better than high breathing. Thirdly there is low breathing or abdominal breathing. This results in higher quality breaths. The fourth type of breath is the complete breath. An aware, slow, steady and deep breath is complete. Imagine your breath coming and going from your navel and tailbone.

All meditation practices note that awareness of breath is essential. All practices similarly point to energy flowing up and down. Your breath travels down the front and instills energy to travel up the back. Every breath you take, every breath of all life on Earth is made up of four parts; inhalation, pause, exhalation, pause. The main polarization is inhalation and exhalation. And as is typical of so many sets of four, often the main polarization is the only one counted. Even though one has breathed for one's entire life one might only notice the main polarization of breath, the inhalation and exhalation. Yet there are four parts to every breath according to longstanding meditation practices in which awareness of breath is essential. The pause full and the pause empty are the second polarity of breath and are just as important to understand.

Meditative breathing requires awareness. Those who practice meditation are taught to be calmly aware of the four parts of breath. Sometimes one or another part is accentuated or lengthened, sometimes a more cyclical breath is utilized and the pauses might be minimized. For balanced deep breathing, noting and often accentuating the pauses is invigorating and beneficial. When performing balanced breathing a ratio of around 4 to 1 seconds seems to be a simple reduction for inhalations/exhalations to pauses. For example seek to breathe in and out for eight second segments and then pause empty and pause full for two seconds. The pause full should be done at around 80 - 85% lung capacity and pause empty at near 0% capacity. Breathing, the essential basis of all life, the beginning to all meditation and action is based a set of four exchanging contrasts of one.

There are innumerable variations of meditative breathing, so many in fact that perhaps awareness of breath is the primary lesson. Despite all variations there are four aspects to all forms of meditative breath. Awareness or consciousness of breath is the first aspect. Slow breath is secondarily important. Thirdly is breathing deeply, down along the spine, from below the navel and ultimately so deep you imagine the breath being drawn through the legs and feet. Lastly is steadiness of breath. This steadiness can fluctuate. Realization of the four parts to every breath and the four aspects to breathing is a simple beginning to heightening awareness of breath, developing one's meditation.

In chi gung, aside from equal and steady breathing, there are four basic breathing forms. Unlike balanced breathing, these forms build or release energy in a certain way. These breaths utilize elongated pauses. The breath form of inhale/pause full/exhale is for Yin energy. The second form, inhale/exhale/pause empty is for Yang energy. Thirdly is inhale/pause/inhale/exhale, which heightens Yin and lastly inhale/exhale/pause/exhale heightening Yang. One can accentuate the pause for however long you can without straining or as the expression goes until 'just before you begin to make yourself angry.'

Chi gung practices also illustrate four pathways of energy through our energy systems; small circle or microcosmic, big circle or macrocosmic, the crossing of the small and the crossing of the big. Chi gung is one of the oldest and original meditative movements and yet also one of the most integrated of perhaps any type of meditative movement. Chi gung has some of simplest, most integrated and alternatively most powerful movements and complex ideas.

In tai chi and chi gung practices there are also two other main aspects of each inhalation and each exhalation. Imagine firstly inhaling into your lower belly and secondly into your lungs, and exhale out of your lungs then lower belly. A variation to this breath is concentration on expanding the lower belly on inhalation and contracting on exhalation, called Buddhist breathing. And alternatively Taoist breathing is contraction of the lower belly on inhalation and expansion on exhalation.

Another breathing technique which is contrary to most mainstream thinking is to breathe unconsciously, to throw out all conceptualization and concentration on breath and to just breathe. In order to breathe unconsciously or as unconsciously as possible breathe though each nostril and your mouth at the same time. Putting your tongue on the roof of your mouth will enable this. Try to breathe from certain points along your spine. You can try breathing in small shallow puffs being sure to make noise. This breath is done slowly and shallowly. The theory behind this is that inhalation is an act of tension, exhalation is an act of relaxation. The less tension is involved with breathing the more relaxation and healing can occur. These short puffs and unconscious breathing in total can help heal and release tension.

There are many ways to breathe and many ways to activate energy, none are wrong and many are exceptional for certain circumstances. Other techniques involving breathing through a particular nostril or in more defined time periods all have different purposes for building energy and concentration in different ways, but are all designed to develop awareness of slow, steady, deep breath. Relaxed awareness is the point of meditation and conversely enhances meditation.

There is plenty to think about and be aware of relevant to each and every breath. At first it might be a stretch to focus on breathing, but eventually one can perform the different types of breathing in a relaxed state. When one settles in meditation the idea is to first focus on breathing so that the distractions of thoughts and emotions do not take over the pursuit of a quality mind state. Thinking of one thing, optimally the breath, enables one to think of nothing, which in turn enables one to ponder all, infinity, like the metaphysical number 108. Concentration on the breath is for the purpose of clearing distracting thoughts and emotions. Once you have mastered clearing distractions you don't need to concentrate on breathing. Thinking of 1 thing, enables thinking nothing, which in turn enables connection with the infinite.

"The fish trap exists because of the fish. Once you've gotten the fish you can forget the trap. The rabbit snare exists because of the rabbit. Once you've gotten the rabbit, you can forget the snare. Words exist because of meaning. Once you've gotten the meaning, you can forget the words. Where can I find a man who has forgotten words so I can talk with him?" ~Zhuangzi

Buddhist and Hindu ideas elaborate on four stages of meditation or four stages of absorption called the four dhyanas. The first dhyana is reached when one releases passions and worldly desires. The second dhyana is reached when the chatter of the intellect is quieted and replaced with single pointed joy. In the third stage the joy fades and is replaced by total equanimity. In the fourth stage all sensation stops and only active equanimity remains.

For best meditations sit or lie down in a comfortable position, but not too comfortable. Many Tibetan lamas and monks do not have beds in the traditional sense. They rest and meditate in cubicles. The boxes allow them to lean against the wall or rest in other positions, but they cannot lie down. Legends about masters of the internal arts going without sleep are common and practitioners often experience needing less sleep. Most meditations remind one to close one's eyes or have them almost all the way closed. Alternatively there are some meditations which prescribe holding the eyes open, so as to focus on being present. This is best done when you are more isolated. Meditation is not sleeping and it is not exactly being awake. Meditation can be compared to the transition period from waking to sleeping, only for a prolonged time period instead of momentary.

Sit down cross legged, sit in a chair or on the edge of a chair or lie down flat on your back. The idea is to be completely still if possible. You can also stand or walk, but these are more physically demanding meditations. Even sitting still cross legged can be physical and yet it becomes easier the more you practice. Try to relax and unclench tension in the muscles and sinews. As you breathe imagine opening up you're your energy fields, chakras, glands and organs. Imagine energy building and opening up from your root chakra, into your sacral chakra, into the solar plexus chakra, continuing up to your heart chakra, then your throat chakra, third eye, and crown. Imagine there is an energy cord connecting you, through your crown chakra, to the macrocosm of the universal energy. Imagine these energies just slightly mixing. Meditative movement activates the mind in certain ways and soon you don't require the movements to activate the mind. All you require is the mind.

Meditate on your breath. Your breath reflects your consciousness which is boundless just as the macrocosmic universes is boundless. Your breath is the microcosmic reflection of your boundless connection to the macrocosm. Eventually, after meditating on one thing, the breath and nothing else, you will on ultimately be able to meditate on nothing at all. And being able to completely silence the chatter of the mind allows consciousness to contemplate anything of the boundlessness. Think of 108, a metaphysically magical number. Meditation on 1 thing allows meditation on 0 things which in turn allows contemplation on anything.

Meditate for five minutes or less, just meditate often. Meditate on being aware, relaxed, peaceful and positive. Meditate on being calm. Meditate on being well. Meditate on simply being and on being simple. Meditate on one single thought or no thought at all. Take a moment when you are sitting at work or sitting on your way to work to meditate. Meditation can be performed while sitting a chair and at any time really.

Perhaps the easiest way to begin a meditation practice is to meditate before you sleep. Do so by lying down flat on your back with your hands cupped (right on top for men, left on top for women) resting on your lower belly or wherever they are comfortable. Lying on the floor is preferable, but the bed works. Bring your knees up so that your feet are resting flat on the surface you're lying on. The trick to meditation is to meditate, just as the trick to walking somewhere is to lift your feet. Everyone has a trickster within that can convince us not to begin. It's the shadow or the ego and the chatter of the mind telling you not to go, all you have to do is start walking.

Sometimes after a rewarding and relaxing meditation session I will be so relaxed, so conscious, that the trickster tries to find ways to be relevant by activating concerns or worry. The trickster or ego or what have you can be so disturbed by the meditative mind state that when I begin to settle back this part of me will literally press the old standby panic buttons and ask, "Wait, where are the keys? And what about your wallet? Aren't you late?" Do not let your ego eliminate the meditative mind state when you gain it. Take the ego and let it go. And worse do not let that part of your mind trick you into not beginning meditation at all.

Meditation benefits circulation, is good for the heart, increases response time, enhances empathy and improves observational skills. It makes you happier and more graceful and makes your happiness less penetrable and your grace less distractible. Meditation has been proven to assist in breaking addiction, cure depression, alleviate stress, improve the ability to maintain calmness in stressful environments, ease chronic pain, cure insomnia and even reduce the blood sugar level of diabetics. Meditation can slow the aging process as well.

Awareness of breath is possibly the most important aspect of meditation. There are many forms of meditation practice that coordinate different abdominal movements with different breathing techniques mindsets all like different keys to different doors to the same building. However all forms of meditation contain the following primordial elements. There are four parts of every breath; inhalation, pause full (~85% capacity), exhalation and pause empty. Take a second or two to be in the pauses. Being attentive of a breath cycles of about 8 seconds inhalation/exhalation and 2 seconds pause full/pause empty is a good way to begin to be aware of and slow the breath. There are also four basic aspects of meditative breathing no matter the variation; breathing slowly, steadily, deeply and consciously. One trick to focus on the breath is to bring your attention to one point. In the beginning of practicing focus on the tip of your nose where the breath originates, as you meditate more or for longer focus your attention on your diaphragm. Try to imagine breathing not from your lungs, but from below you belly button.

Meditation rids one of tension however it is sometimes important to actively bring about a relaxed state as one meditates. One must actively quiet and relax the mind, body and breath. The shoulders are stressed the most among men and the hips for women, both hold tension in the chin and shins. Think about relaxing the tension you are aware of and think about relaxing the tension you are accustomed to and do not notice as much because of the long term presence. Think about ridding yourself of thoughts which can contribute to or be outright causational of tension. Such thoughts might be immediately recognizable as such and others might have accompanied you for so long they might be harder to find.

The mental and physical benefits of meditation are numerous and include renewed vitality of body and mind in multiple ways. The spiritual benefits of meditation are incalculably many. Life is often comparable to a series of peaks and valleys, some more extreme than others. As you traverse the peaks and valleys the mind will always try to maintain its control. When you are high the mind will induce the idea that you do not need to practice your meditation for everything is already wonderful. When you are low the mind will focus on the idea that you do need to practice meditation for it has not helped in any great way to alleviate the current predicament in a shady valley. Do not let the mind maintain control. Open up to consciousness through meditation. Meditation always uplifts.

When time and circumstances permit, after you have meditation experience and after you have practiced Tibetan Fusion or some other series of meditative movements for a while, do your chores while performing meditative movements intermittently. It is preferable that you have some isolation while you clean or do the dishes or whatever it is that you or others consider the gritty and dirty work and then mix in your meditation. Clean for five or ten minutes and then meditate for about the same time or do a project for five or ten minutes and then mix in your meditation project for the same time. Doing this occasionally can subtly heighten meditation experience and allow integration of the meditative mind state into daily activities.

Ideally meditative movement should be done prior to meditation. And though meditation can be done without being preceded by meditative movement, meditative movement should always end with and be topped by still meditation. Meditative movement is like driving a vehicle. Meditation is shutting down the vehicle properly. And meditation is your destination.

Simple directions for meditation:

Find quiet.

Find a comfortable, but not too comfortable, position.

Find inner quiet, peace and think compassionate thoughts for yourself, others, the joy of others and all things.

Think of being grounded to the core of the planet and imagine starlight coming through you as you are grounded.

Relax tension.

Concentrate on your breath.

Be present.

Be still.

Be happy.

Let thoughts/emotions come and go like waves.

Focus on complete clearness. Or focus on solving whatever problem might be at hand. Never focus on social wants/needs. Focus on nothing or something of depth.

Slow the breath.

General Rules for Meditative Movements

Practice for an hour or more a day. Practicing for ten minutes a day is of course enormously better than no practice. The morning is the best time to practice for most people. Try to make your practice a routine. Repeat a movement done with one side the same number of times with the other side using the same amount of force, speed, size, time and so on. Think of slow, steady and aware movements. Never cause yourself pain, know the difference between strain and pain. Never lock your joints and ligaments. Even when you are in a position requiring one be straight always have your legs and arms just slight bent and just slightly loosened. Never lock your ligaments, especially the knees and elbows.

The point is to open up so think about being soft and pliable even when exerting tremendous energy. The point is to gain strength through elimination of rigidity. Such softness in tai chi is compared to being a paper bag or towel. One cannot damage a paper bag or towel by punching it. It absorbs every blow. One should be loose as a paper bag so that impacts for instance are absorbed and belittled.

It is especially important to do certain aspects of Tibetan Fusion as described. For instance try to do the joint rotation movements, the Eight Brocades and the Five Tibetan Rites of Rejuvenation in their entirety when you do them. However each of these series of movements can be done on their own independently. Tibetan Fusion works well as a series done in the following order, but you can make your own alterations or additions or some parts can be removed to manage time or what have you. The idea of floor stretching, standing stretching, primal loosening, breath work and meditative movement leading into the more vigorous Five Tibetan Rites of Rejuvenation and meditation is the main order of operations that is important to consider.

In meditative movement classes the first thing you will learn is to loosen up. Relax and let go. The point is to loosen up. Be free. Do not allow rigidity to form for such leads to hardness which develops into tension which can lead to inflammation and ultimately injury and illness. Tension is next to restriction and can be factor in inflammation. Relaxation is next to integration and leads to wellbeing. Be free, loose and open. Adopt and integrate the practices you learn as your own.

Tibetan Fusion

1. To begin kneel on a yoga mat or floor with a rug. Cross your big toes together if comfortable. Relax in this position for a moment or a minute or two, longer if you like. Tibetan Fusion allows room, it is open to your unique flow. If kneeling is too painful try it sitting on a yoga block or with a folded up blanket between your legs and buttock. Slow down the breath and then release thoughts and stresses. Be thankful for your practice and your devotion to it. Think about straightening your back.

When you are ready inhale your left arm up and press your right palm down on the floor and gently bend to the right. Alternate to the left and repeat once or up to three times. Look over the left shoulder and then the right for awakening slight twist. Bring your arms to your side or in front of you if you require a little more support and bow forward on exhalation aiming to press your third eye into the floor keeping your back straight. Rise in a ready and relaxed manner. Do once or repeat up to three times. Eventually you will be able to bend forward without any support, your arms aside you or cupping your ankles.

If kneeling is out of the question just sit cross legged and loosen up your mind by slowing down your breathing and loosen up your body however feels appropriate. And think of straightening your back. Or just go straight into Child's pose.

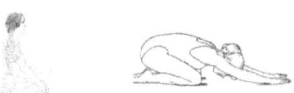

2. Go into child's pose by spreading your knees, but keeping your big toes together. Bringing your forearms in front of you and elongating your back by pressing your palms onto the floor. Remain in this position to lengthen your back and slow your breath. At you're pace rise up onto our palms, knees and balls of your feet so your palms are below your shoulders and knees below your hips. Take a few cat breaths inhaling and arching the back so you are looking upward and exhale rounding the back looking downward.

When ready after 3 to 6 cat breaths, on an inhalation stand up to your big toes and palms using your hands to walk forward to form an upside down V with your body, knees bent, unlocked. Relax and loosen your legs by pressing and unweighting your feet as you walk your ankles around, up and down, one at time and together. When you're ready walk your feet and palms together and prepare to stand up. Bring your feet together, toes and ankles touching or wider if needed for more stability, then on an inhalation rise so that your back is parallel with the ground, hands pressing on your shins, head relaxed looking down. Take a few breaths to elongate your back this way. Rise to standing on an inhalation and try to keep your back straight.

3. Stand straight and relaxed and practice the bone tapping/tai chi technique of rotating on one's axis or ringing the bell. Relax and make sure your knees are rooted, but unlocked. This basic warm up builds energy through the gentle rotation of your spine and from it its simplicity sprouts man more complex tai chi movements. Imagine as if you were armless and the action was originating in your dantien, the space just below your belly button where according many traditions all movement and energy originates, the root chakra. As you go imagine the movement is originating in your grounded feet and continuing through your loose knees and hips. Rotate back and forth and keep facing straight ahead. Stand with your feet touching. The concept is to keep your weight together on foot or, most easily with your feet touching. After doing it this way you can shift your weight as you go or change how they are touching, next to each other or one on top of the other. When you stand with your feet apart make sure practically all your weight remains on one foot as you go or one foot shifting weight from foot to foot. No matter the variation try to root yourself, connect with the ground through the balls of your feet. Tap the lower back and the kidneys lightly with your arms as you rotate. Further imagine your chi is moving you with your arms swinging low.

The same movement can be done only with more swinging power so that your hands end up tapping heart, lungs and collarbone area. Then after swinging mid power to tap the mid area use even more swinging power and tap your back behind your shoulders. The same principles apply. Imagine tapping and moving all stagnate stress with the relaxed weight of yourself. Ringing the bell in low, mid and high forms is extremely beneficial to opening up old injuries and moving energy. The low format is the most important of the three forms.

Martial artists frequently use an alternate variation of this movement by initiating harder strikes onto their bodies hitting their chest, back and ultimately their collarbone too by more forcefully dropping their weight onto themselves with relaxed but heavy hands. This harder form can be used for energy and internal development, but is not necessary.

Relaxation and removal of stagnation is the goal and one need not exert much, if any force at all. Low bell ringing is the most important, though all are work well.

Ringing the bell is one of the original, most fundamental and most valuable warming and loosening movements. It is a primal movement, as are many body movements. You will note many young children performing this and other such movements as if instinctually building chi or warming themselves.

Look at your palms before doing Tibetan Fusion, tai chi or chi gung or just the axis rotational bone tapping of bell ringing. Then look at them after ten to twenty minutes of practice and throughout the meditative movement process to see indicators of chi movement. Look at them after other forms of exercise to compare. Chi is visible and eventually felt as tingling or pulsing in the palms. One will see one's palms go from one a uniform color to splotchy. The more intense the white splotches, the more chi is moving. The splotches that develop on the palms are from blood flow and chi flow increase.

Ringing the bell can be done anytime, while not necessarily practicing, or during practice as one feels it necessary to take a breath or feels the need to stir up energy and shake out the body. I suggest doing it intermittently through practice as you feel you need to.

4. When you're ready stop ringing the bell. On an inhalation, while looking straight ahead raise your arms from your sides too prayer above your head then bow toward the ground in a forward fold on the exhalation. Reach for a comfortable stretch to your shins or ankles or feet or placing your palms on the floor and ultimately intending to put your head between your knees. Rise on the inhalation so your arms are in prayer position above then repeat a total of three times.

A variation of forward fold can be done in combination with a beck bend by placing your hands on your lower back on your and bowing from standing, on the exhale, without reaching for floor then rising and bending backward. Another form can utilize the arms to reach for the ground as you fold forward and reach up when you bend back always inhaling up and exhaling down. This can be done with the feet together or shoulder width.

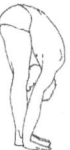

5. Step your feet out as wide as your arms wing span so your ankles are about under your wrists. Reach your arms out to your sides. Keeping your body in line gently fold over so that your right palm presses you're the outside of your right shin with the left reaching up. Imagine widening yourself. Switch sides and repeat a total of three times or more if you desire. Now bend forward and press the left palm onto the floor and bring the right arm up, palm open, vertically in line with the left arm while twisting and looking up. Alternate sides and repeat the same number of times.

   Without straining your knees, keeping them just slightly bent and unlocked, lean forward onto the palms of your hands and walk forward on your hands to elongate your back while looking downward. In this position you can lengthen and straighten your back. Adjust your legs and hands for comfort and be in this position with as little tension as possible. The main idea is to lengthen your back. Being parallel to the ground is not important. Try to relax in this position and only go as far as is comfortable. Rise when you're ready by inching your legs together, walking back with your hands and pushing yourself upright.

6. Back opener. With a walking stick or utilizing your hands to press on your bent knees, standing with your feet about shoulder width apart, bend forward so that your back is completely straight and parallel with the ground. You can relax and straighten out your neck as well so that it is nearly straight along with you back. Enjoy this position. Elongate the back and allow opening in the process. Assistance of a mirror is helpful for this in the beginning. See what you think is straight then have someone adjust or look in the mirror. Utilize holding the walking stick to stretch out your shoulders and back.

7. Standing fold to the floor to handstand. Bring your feet parallel to each other about shoulder width apart. On inhalation raise hands up above your head to prayer and bow down on exhalation head following hands, bending the knees and pressing your palms onto the floor in front of your feet. Stay in this position for a few breaths, then further bend your legs, engage your upper body so as to balance on your palms with weight pressing all the way onto the extended fingertips. With your palms pressing on the ground, elbows unlocked, knees slightly bent, bend your knees more, rise onto your toes and press your body weight through your knees into your arms and lift your feet off of the ground while looking down. Remain balanced in this position as long as you are able to upper body strength. If you are able, cross your legs while holding this position on your palms and allow yourself to settle into a seated cross legged position on the floor. You can simply sit into a squat position and then sit back if you are unable to settle into cross legged sitting position

from handstand. This is the easiest handstand to do, but nonetheless, be careful not to push forward and over.

8. Take a moment toward meditative mindset and clear the breathing/energy channels. Bring yourself into cross legged position or any lotus variation, sitting upright with your back straight. Meditate for a moment with your eyes open or closed.

If you want to practice burning a tear you can now. In order to burn a tear hold your eyes open and do not blink. Focus on a single point in front of you, a candle or something in the distance or even a point on a wall. Keep your eyes open until, ideally, each releases one tear or try. Afterwards cover your eyes and rotate your pupils equally and move them diagonally, side to side and up and down, equally. Whether you feel like burning a tear or not simply try to relax and slowdown your breath. Think about loosening any clenching or tightness.

In this cross legged position rotate your lower back and abdomen clockwise and then counterclockwise. Rotate your shoulders the same and then your neck. Be gentle and careful with your neck. Three to nine rotations in each direction is sufficient.

Return to a straight position and tuck your tailbone in a little. Inhale you abdomen in, your buttocks up and straighten your back. Bring your forefingers to touch your thumbs and extend your other three fingers. Rest them on your knees and meditate on your back being straight.

Men use the right hand, women left. Change your right hand position so that you pinky and ring finger are pointing straight and you middle and pointer fingers are bent down with your thumb out. Place your right thumb over the right nostril and inhale, exhale with your right ring finger covering your left nostril. Then keep your fingers on your nostril and inhale then switch on the exhale. Repeat this alternating process for sixth breaths. Women begin with the alternate side and then proceed in the same manner. When one has the time you can separately do this alternating breathing for ten to thirty minutes as a powerful meditation all on its own.

9. Hip opening. Remain sitting. Bring you left foot to your right thigh with your right leg straight. Stretch by pressing knee toward floor and rotating/adjusting ankle as you need. Be aware of straightening your back so it's perpendicular to the floor. Repeat in the same manner with the same force on the right side. Repeat as you like, three or more times. This asana or position can be done whenever, even just after eating. This asana stretches and

opens the hips, knees and ankles and practicing the position will allow you to eventually go into full locked lotus if that is a goal.

Next are sitting tree and forward folds. Bring your left foot to your right inner thigh in a bow position. Start with your hands at your sides. On the inhalation raise your straight arms above your head slowly turning your palms in the process so that they together in prayer directly above your head with arms straight. Bend forward on the exhalation, keep your leg straight. Go as far as is comfortable, just keep your leg straight. Hold for a breath or two. Repeat total of three times. Switch sides and do the same.

Now stretch in the same manner with both feet in front of you. There are numerous variations and at times competing theories describing the manner in which to perform this particular stretch. I believe the main idea is not to pain or even strain yourself. You can grab your toes, ankles or knees depending on your flexibility. Try to straighten your back while looking straight ahead. In contrast some say to bring your head to your knees with the intention to look downward at the floor between the knees. Do both; the first variation for a breath or three and the second for the same amount of time or less. You can, in either of these positions, rock from side to side, just to the point of teetering, while holding onto your toes or feet, adding movement in a slow and relaxed manner.

Then bring both legs apart two to four feet depending on your flexibility and while pressing your body into the floor press your forearms in front of you. Hold this position the same amount of time as the other forward folds or longer if it suits you.

Rise and straighten your back. When ready inhale your palms to prayer and bring to your sternum. On exhalation reach your hands in between your feet. Relax in the position, not reaching as far as possible, but just being.

Now for the bow position bring both feet together in front of you so that the soles of the feet are touching and form a diamond like shape in front of you. On exhalation, bend forward with the intention of touching your toes to the center of your forehead. On inhalation rise so your back is vertical. Hold and/or repeat total of three times. It is more important to be free, hold and repeat as you like, only move in coordination with the breath.

10. Rocking. Keep your feet in this position, soles of the feet touching. On inhalation bring your arms to prayer position to the crown of your head. On inhalation allow yourself to fall backwards rolling on your back. On the exhalation roll back up and bend forward so that your head touches your toes. Repeat three to six times. If this move is too much warm up to it by lying down and bringing your feet up to you and grabbing your toes and then rocking

back and forth and around in this position. If you can't grab your toes embrace your knees and rock around the same way side to side being mind to lengthen the back so your tailbone is in contact with the floor.

11. Lower back opening series. Set your feet down and then together and let the legs relax into a bow position while lying on your back with your hands at your sides. Hold for as long as you like and allow gravity to stretch out your hips and lower back.

Now set your feet down on the floor with your knees bent and your arms at your sides palms down on the ground. On an inhalation slowly lift your back beginning with the tailbone, imagining lifting on vertebrae at a time smoothly and steadily so that you end up with most of your weight on the soles of your feet and shoulders. And when you return to the floor, on exhalation, try to slowly set each vertebrae down one after the other, slowly. Repeat three or six times.

Set your legs down and bring your arms above your head resting on the floor palms up. While lying down reach this way reach with the left toes and left hand so as to lengthen completely on an inhale and release on exhale. Do the same on the right side. Now do the same with the left toes and right hand and next the right toes and left hand. Now relax. Take a breath or two and on an exhalation utilizing your arms above your head to assist sit up. Extend your legs apart and in front of you, the more limber you are the wider you can go. Adjust the width so that you can bend forward on the exhalation and press your forearms onto the floor in front you. Rise on the inhalation and repeat three breaths, then hold for several breaths.

12. Twists are important parts of any regimen. Lift left knee up into a triangle position and set the sole of the foot on the floor over the other leg. Set the right leg the leg into triangle also only remaining on the floor. Set your right arm across your knee to grab your toes then look to the left. Hold for thirty seconds or more and repeat the other way.

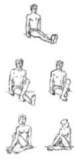

Bend both legs into triangle position and set one on top of the one set on the floor. Look straight ahead with your back straight and erect. Grab the toes of corresponding hands.

Then grab the alternate toes, left with right, right with left. Then perform the same on the alternate side for balance.

13. Shake it out. From cross legged position with your right arm gently slap your left shoulder and slide down to the wrist, then alternate sides. Unravel both legs and wipe both at the same time in the same manner and then bend forward and exhale stale air from your mouth. Shake your wrists. The hands are loosened up in the beginning so they can release and exchange energy. With your feet in front of you shake your wrists more. Bend your knees and lift your ankles grabbing them from above the joint on the inside of the legs and shake them too. Let go of the tension holding the ankles and wrists and allow movement. The idea is to loosen the joints. Keep on shaking your ankles when you let go of them and shake your wrists along with them variously in front of you and above your shoulders.

You can shake it up standing too. Rise up and down on your feet as if huffing. Shake your wrists, hands, shoulders, chest, back, abdomen, hips and knees. Imagine shaking out tension, restriction and inflammation with movement and relaxation. Allow yourself to move unrestricted by form. As you shake integrate tapping your heels to tap the floor sending slight vibrations through the body. Such primal shaking fires off muscles and creates the ability for a fast twitch response later. This type of freestyle shaking is frequently incorporated into chi gung practice.

In a more controlled manner swing your arms around in circles one at a time in both directions while the other hand is at your sternum is prayer position. The circles should be done determinedly, but should be relaxed loose swinging. Do nine circles in each direction and slowly increase the number of circles, up to a hundred repetitions.

14. Cross legged warm up. The Tibetans believe that hopping from cross legged position is the first step to levitation. The Tibetans originally used straw under a deer skin for this and similar practices, the original yoga mat. A soft cushion or yoga mat on top of rug or two yoga mats or whatever you see as appropriate is fine. With practice beginning Tibetan monks were able to pass a test of hopping out of a hole dug into the ground. A sandy beach or similarly dense ground can be ideal, providing rebound to hop off of and cushion to disperse the landing.

To warm up for the Tibetan hopping, if you are able, sit in lotus position with your legs locked or sit in a simple cross legged position. Now, use the strength of your shoulders to push yourself up onto your palms or fingertips and drop so that your tailbone and lower back are stimulated by the small drop onto your behind. If you are able lift yourself farther up with a full inhalation (80% -85% lung capacity) using the strength of your shoulders to rise onto your fingertips, do so and drop the same on the exhale. If you are able to hold yourself up for a moment or minute, do so, and on an exhalation drop with a noticeable exhale. To integrate energy when you drop, bring your hands up to touch your shoulders, so that your elbows point out to the sides. You can do the same thing without having your legs locked and without bringing your hands to your shoulders.

Then from an unlocked cross legged position with feet set slightly more narrow together than usual rise to a standing jump. Rise up with your arms in unison at your sides on an inhalation so that you spring aloft hands pointed straight up and land with your feet straight just under shoulder width. Sit back down repeat 3 or more times and repeat with your feet set in the opposite cross.

Then simply work on hopping up with your feet from a cross legged position. Your arms stay at your sides or you can use your hands to help you hop providing just a slight and subtle push to further the hop along with the feet. Pop into the air and land onto your buttock and lower back. This taps the root chakra and energizes the feet and legs. The vibrations can also reduce tension along the spine and in the ribcage. Use your hands in combination with your feet or just your feet to hop and vibrate through the tailbone or root chakra. An inch or less is enough, but you can go higher with practice. Exhale on the impact so as to relax and allow the vibrations to move tension.

Following practicing and understanding these variations expand on them with this one. Sit cross legged with one leg just on top of the other with so that that foot can easily press onto the ground. Bring your hands to your upper thighs with your hands making the shape of a gun, though the three fingers are bent and folded at the knuckle above complete fist closure, with the pointer out and without clenching. Press down with the backs of your hands on your legs so that your arms are straight or near straight and point to each other on inhalation. Hold position and breath for a moment. Now from the cross legged position spring up a couple inches or more and land on you buttock. Do so with an exclamation during exhalation, 'Hai!' or other syllable more meaningful to you, setting your hands at your sides, palms open at 45 degrees in unison. Repeat this three or more times breathing out loudly on impact if with an audible exclamation. Repeat with the alternate leg positioning.

Experienced Tibetan yogis learn numerous variations of this simple exercise which stimulates and the root chakra and sends energy upward. Experienced practitioners of trul khor and/or or tsa lung can literally jump from half lotus multiple feet into the air then in midair lock to full lotus before returning to the ground. Another variation is hopping rapidly at a jogger's pace while in full lotus. Do not attempt these.

15. Tai chi squats. Do not do these if you have recent knee or leg injuries or if they hurt. Sit down with your legs crossed. Enjoy the energy you are awakening. Meditate for a moment with your hands on your knees palms up or momentarily press the backsides of the wrists onto the inner thighs for wrist stretch and so as to adjust and straighten the back before setting hands on knees. Set your feet crossed set slightly narrower than you would normally have them. When ready, on inhalation rise and twist a full 360. Utilize your hands if necessary to initiate the upward thrust. Eventually synchronize the breath and the rising with raising the hands at your sides so they are above your head when you are reach upright position, you can interlace the fingers or bring them into prayer position, and set the arms back down as you exhale and sit. Return straight down to the floor, again utilizing the hands if necessary and moving slowly and steadily in coordination with the breath. When done correctly (don't think about it and it will happen naturally) you will end up facing the same way as were sitting down only your legs will be crossed differently. Now do the same again, only this time you will naturally rotate in the other direction because of how your feet are now set. Repeat at least three times each side. Take a moment to meditate and breathe in cross legged position after doing them and then stand and up again and adjust to normal upright position.

If the twisting tai chi squats are too much you can try rising straight up from the cross legged position. Bring your feet in just slightly narrower than usual in cross legged position. On an inhalation shoot straight up including a small jump and raise your hands above your head to point up with one or two fingers landing on the balls of your feet, if you can, looking up if you can.

If this is too much simply squat, always mindful to go slow and never position your knees beyond your toes and always in line with your ankles. Think about beginning with slow squats being more important than deep squats. With your feet at about shoulder width apart perform the motion of sitting only do not sit, pause, as if you are sitting, if you are able. Extend your hands in front of you for counter balance and allow your body to come back to rest on your heels to the point where your toes lift slightly.

Another movement you can incorporate at this point whether or not you are able to do the tai chi squats or not is standing on one leg. The simplest way is to stand with your hands at your hips and just lift your leg so that your thigh is parallel with the floor. A tai chi and chi gung variation of this is to begin in this static position and then allow the leg without weight on it to move into different positions, more or less freely.

Another variation to develop leg strength and balanced concentration is called the tree. This position is done by lifting the sole of the foot to the opposite thigh, above the knee and bringing your hands to prayer at your sternum or even opening arms above your head like branches. Important: do not rest the foot on knee in the tree pose.

I highly recommend incorporating being in the horse stance for at least a few minutes a day to develop overall leg strength and stability. Stand with your feet wide and sit as if riding a horse. Ultimately you want to sit deeply so that your thighs are parallel with the floor, however start at whatever positioning you are able. Your toes are pointed outward a little and you keep your back straight. Hold this position for a time, the longer the better. Hands in prayer at your sternum can help balance in this position. Be mindful of your knee positioning so they are above the feet or as close to above the feet as possible.

16. Grounding bone tapping series. Perhaps the most primal internal/martial art is bone tapping or patting a form of self-massage. One of the most primal ways to move energy is through this system. These are very simple movements. Rotating one's axis is an example of bone tapping though there are many systems which utilize bone tapping or integrate bone tapping practices. The following series of bone tapping movements integrates aspects of chi gung, tai chi and Tibetan yoga. They are put together in such a way as to be a process that can be utilized by all at any time. They can be done be done with integration of the rest of Tibetan Fusion and they can be done individually.

The principle in combining them in the following manner is to stimulate and root one's mudras and chakras in a uniform way, from essentially the bottom up, following chi gung theory of grounding. As you tap yourself breathe out on the impact so as to allow resonance and elimination of tension. This becomes more important the harder you tap.

Bone tapping is a vigorous and stimulating self-massage. Bone tapping is an excellent way to build energy and eliminate tension. This series works upward having a rooting effect. With legs and above always tap the relaxed limb on which there is no weight, this way the vibration travels deeper and farther. Tap your shins and the muscle just to the outside of your shins with your knuckles or even a stick as many times as you like, between 9 and 36 times. Start with the left shin, with your weight on the right foot. Use the heel of your hand to rub your shins downward about the same number of times imagining moving stagnant chi, the energetic cause of shin splints using the same principle, switch sides utilizing the same principle of tapping the side that is not bearing weight. Tap the sides and backs of your calves forcefully. Tap the back of your knees, left side first, without weight. Repeat the same number of times thereabouts, 9 -36. Next tap the backs of your legs solidly with your palms or fists. Then tap the front of the legs and thighs with the heel of your hand utilizing the same left to right function and the same number of times. Then use the back of your hand to tap your buttocks, your lower back, your tailbone and sacrum as many times as you like. With each hand the same number of times or just both palms massage your organs and abdomen, clockwise and then counterclockwise, 9 to 36 times. Especially rub any spots of tension. Tap you your kidneys in the same way as your tailbone only more gently, 9 times is sufficient. Imagine the tapping releasing soot from your kidneys.

Tap the left back shoulder with your right palm and slide palm down your arm 6 to 36 times. Tap the tops of your shoulder with palm and slide in the same way then more softly the collarbone sliding the same way; as if not only performing physical resonation and energy movement at the same time sliding along the arm with your palm after the tap or palm drop. Then switch to tap the right side. Remember to apply the same strength to each side the same number of times.

Tap your neck your fingers. Lightly tap your jaw. Pull your ear lobes. Tap the crown of your head with you knuckles.

With your middle finger, rub along the sides of the nose, where the nose meets the cheek, 6 times. Rub your forehead side to side the same and face side to side with alternating palms 6 to 12 times. Gently rub your neck from your below your chin to your sternum 6 to 9 times alternating hands using the palms of your hands. Gently rub your face, side to side, up and down, alternating, direction and hands six to nine times with your palms. Use these numbers as general guidelines and perform as many you're comfortable, but never too many.

All sorts of meditative practitioners, chi gung and Tibetan yoga especially it seems, utilze energy washing techniques. The idea is to stimulate the skin, the only organ you can touch, so as to as in moving energy. Energy washing is done by essentially using your palms to make circular movements on the abdomen, chest and back for instance and sliding movements on the appendages. Energy washing can be done firmly, softly and eventually without touching the body. This can be utilized with and/or after bone tapping in the same upward format.

A great way to tap your back and send vibrations throughut your whole body, is to do what I call wall falls. Stand about a foot or less, maybe more, whatever feels comfortable, away from a solid wall, tree or ideally a flat pole and allow yourself to fall back onto it. Exhale out and allow the vibration to travel as your back taps the wall. Allow yourself to variously and gently fall onto your shoulders, upper back and lower back. Allow vibratory effect through landing on muscle and exhaling to move. This process stimulates and generates resonating chi and can be tremendously healing.

17. Stand up to perform joint rotations. Ring the bell for a little bit loosening and rotating on the axis. Perform tai chi joint rotations slowly and steadily and equal rate and size. Imagine this process roots you to the ground as well as opens you up. Meditative movements have direct physical attributes and benefits as well as more subtle spiritual or energetic benefits. The physical mechanics of tai chi rotations loosen tension and bring revived fluid to the sinews of body, the metaphysical mechanics revive the energy points or vortices so they spin at an optimal rate. The idea is not to use force while performing tai chi rotations, but to relax so that micro muscles are used and subtle energy is built. This is a contrast to

Begin with your ankles. Rotate your ankles in a relaxed and focused fashion first clockwise and counterclockwise six times each. Do the same number of rotations with your knees touching and then with your feet slightly under shoulder width apart. (Never put your knees past your toes in tai chi and practically any exercise! Imagine there is a line coming straight up from your big toe. If your knee bends past that adjust so that your knee is closer to being above your ankle rather over your toes.) Do the same number or more rotations with your hips, slowly and intentionally.

You can always rotate your hips more, and should, a minimum of thirty times is decent, smaller and larger circles, each direction. Include another loosening movement by holding your hips and in a relaxed manner swinging your left leg forward and backward three to nine times and then doing the same with the right leg. If you are comfortable and your lower back is not injured you can swivel your hips in another manner by kicking your left knee up and inward while at the same time swinging your arms outward. Alternate and repeat a total of three times.

Rotate your wrists the same way six to nine times, inward circles first. Next are the shoulders. Rotate them, forward first. You can use the palm hand of the arm which is not rotating to stabilize the shoulder and sternum while rotating. You can also lift and shrug your shoulders up and then release them down three times or more imagining energy moving through the feet.

Finally rotate the neck, in extraordinarily small circles, slowly and relaxed, clockwise and counterclockwise. Always be extra gentle and careful with your neck. I close my eyes and mostly move my neck nearly imperceptibly small circles.

18. The Eight Pieces of Brocade. I barely ever teach this in class partly because it takes up a lot of time and is perhaps a class itself, but this is a great way to warm up the legs by maintaining horse stance throughout most of the movements. The eight pieces of silk or eight pieces of brocade has been performed on its own and integrated endlessly in variation. The form is utilized in chi gung and possibly is integrated into some Tibetan forms of yoga as well as Shaolin Kung Fu. It is utilized as a standing practice and there is a sitting meditation with the same name. Like all tai chi and most chi gung the standing Eight Brocades can be done in a relaxed manner, slowly and meditatively, slowly and intensely or more rapidly and intensely.

Begin performing them in a totally relaxed manner. Either way the form is beneficial and can be done by itself as a quick wake up in the morning or all on its own. Repeat each of the Brocades once, three, six, eight, nine, twelve, or twenty-one times, only do each one an equal amount of times.

The Eight Brocades is a perfect example of a set of movements which has been endlessly integrated with other disciplines. The Eight Brocades can be performed utilizing numerous variations in posture and even order of operations and yet it is so simple and effective that it practically cannot be done wrong and can be endlessly honed, bettered, transformed and perfected. They are simple and effective and easily integrated into other practices if not already, either directly or as variations.

The Eight Brocades was originated by a general who watched his army fall apart physically. The Eight Brocades were designed to heal and strengthen through opening up the body that had experienced hostility, horseback riding and hiking in extreme conditions. When practicing one's mindset should be as a warrior in training. The warrior training you are undergoing is not a martial one, but an internal one. You should imagine, when the stance is obviously made for striking that you are striking and destroying bad ideas, stress and the negativity we all experience. Imagine you are battling and defeating the injury or thee very shadow of yourself, your ego. Remember to breathe in coordination with the movement, inhaling on the contraction and exhaling on the relaxation.

#1 Pressing Up to Heaven. Raise your hands above your head with your fingers interlaced on inhalation or the tips just touching. Including a bend from side to side in this position is an important variation. Bring your hands down to an unlaced cupped position at your dantien, fingertips touching or cupped, men with the right hand on top, women the left.

#2 Drawing The Bow and Letting The Arrow Fly. With your hands pointed with one or two fingers pretend to pull open a bow and release an arrow beginning with shooting to the left position then releasing and rotating to the left to pull the bow on the inhalation. You can imagine pulling a large bow of great force in slow motion then shooting an arrow into the infinite or at a target. On the exhalation release and bring your arms to a guard position, forearms next to each other . and rotating to pull again the other direction.

#3 Separating Heaven and Earth. This movement is similar to #1 only you lift one hand to the sky while press the other hand to the ground. Each wrist is active on reaching the top or bottom depending on the alternation each pointed inward.

#4 The Wise Owl Looks Backward. This one presents a series of easy twists. Stand with your feet shoulder width apart with your hands at your sides. While maintaining a straight back look to each side and upwards only moving your neck. With your right arm palm up and extended to the left and reach up and behind, alternate sides. Look to each side with your hands at your abdomen fingers touching. Then twist to each side with your hands interlaced behind your back. Do each the same number of times.

#5 Big Bear Bends from Side to Side. With your hands on your needs rotate about 270 degrees, beginning in a clockwise direction as if a powerful bear. Alternate sides.

#6 Touching The Toes and Bending Backwards. With your arms lifted gently above your head reach up and back on the inhalation. On exhalation reach down to your feet and pull up your toes.

#7 Lifting The Pillar. With your feet together and arms at your side on an inhalation rise up onto the tips of your toes and bring your arms up, bending from the elbows so that your fists face each other at your belly, with your forearms parallel with the floor. Repeat.

#8 Punching With an Angry Glare. Begin with your hands at your sides in horse stance with your palms facing up in fists. Punch forward on the exhalation with your left fist unraveling and rotating the fist so that it is upright just as you near the end of the blow. Alternate doing the same on the right side. Now punch to the left side using the same rotating unraveling peaking on the end of blow. Repeat on the right side. These four blows equal one set of #8. When you have finished however many sets you are doing raise you fists to the left, your palms facing you, with your right hand lower and behind your left. Breathe in this position for a bit imagining facing off whatever your foe may be, be it an inner demon or an actual tormentor in the form of a person or an adversarial affliction. Switch sides and face the right in the same manner with the same mindset. With each punch think of expelling some of the energy you just summoned doing the Eight Brocades so that the energy is moving and not just simply building.

The sitting Eight Brocades is much more meditative and focused on establishing inner rhythms with much more subtle movements, though some variations of the sitting Eight Brocades contain similar aspects to the standing series. I will occasionally perform a variation of the physical movements of the Eight Brocades, while sitting cross legged, as a way to warm up. I will often include some bone patting, energy washing and Tibetan hopping before or after. Sometimes I will perform all the Eight Brocades in the horse stance. Being in the horse stance for any length of time will develop core leg strength.

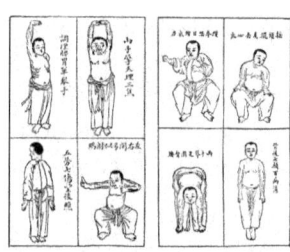

19. Tai chi rocking and standing breathwork. This exercise betters balance and stimulates chi flow. Begin by standing with feet shoulder width apart. On the inhalation bring your hands, fingers facing up just in front of you and lift your heels about an inch, your weight on your toes. On the exhalation bring your hands downward just behind your hips, lifting your toes and put your weight on your heels. You can remember the hand positioning through holding tea cups on the inhale and cat clawing on exhale. Repeat the rocking motion for as long as you like, at least a couple of minutes. As you develop this movement you can then vary. Do the opposite movement with your hands; when you are on your toes bring them just behind you and when you are on your heels bring them in front of you. Never put your knees past your toes. This is a standing meditation, remember to be meditative, moving slowly in coordination with the breath.

There are many variations of tai chi breathing, or standing meditations. Stand your feet straight about shoulder width apart. Cup your hands together, right hand on top for men, left hand on top for women. Hold your hands at you waist. Imagine that there is a ball of glowing energy emanating from you. On the inhalation lift your hands up and caress the energy ball so that when you have taken a full breath your hands are now facing downward. On exhalation return to the starting position. Repeat this for a few minutes at least.

To expand on this movement bring your feet to slightly wider than shoulder width. On inhalation keep raising your hands, bring your hands together in prayer at your face and continue so until they reach straight up above the head and then open them to your sides, like a lotus flower.

On exhalation reverse the movement. Bring your hands back to prayer, extended straight above your head, then bring your arms downward, hands remaining in prayer. Follow your hands, in other words do not start bending your back until your hands bring there. Dive forward, bending your back so that your prayer hands touch the floor or reach back behind your legs. Repeat three to six times.

Now with your feet shoulder width apart or a little wider and hands at your waist level arms facing down and hands just in front of you, breathe in. On exhalation gently press all your weight into your left leg and swivel your gaze and your palms to where you're looking downward at your left foot. Inhale and then on the exhalation slide your hands to the right and your weight into the right foot. Inhale while still and exhale while moving your hands, weight and gaze to the left. Repeat for a few minutes.

I always like to ring the bell a little after breathing slowly and steadily for any length of time. Ringing the bell is a great way to loosen up at any time and is important to do as a way to stir up energy you just awakened around.

In creating energy for your use it is just as important to dissipate the energy as it is to build the energy. This is why the corpse position is used to end a series of movements so as to allow the energy to settle. This is why so many of the most primal meditative movements have components f wiping the energy off of them or closing down the system you just revved up, similar to ending a car drive. You must take off your seatbelt, put on the brake, turn off the ignition and then get out of the car. In healing arts healers consider closing and settling after healing. Ringing the bell and tapping wherever you feel is necessary is a great way to stir and ultimately help settle energy, in balance.

20. Perform the Five Tibetan Rites of Rejuvenation. Be sure to do each Rite the same number of times. Start at 3, 6, 9, 12 or whatever number you feel comfortable with. Start with 3 or 6 if you are injured or unaccustomed to yoga and physical activity. Each Rite should be performed the same number of times for balance, as with any such set of movements. 21 repetitions is considered the optimal number of repetitions for the Rites. The idea behind these meditative movements is that they activate the proper spinning of the chakras which spin clockwise. With intention one can eventually do 21 with ease or more. Doing more repetitions will give you more of a physical workout, but 21 times moves the energy properly. Doing more repetitions may be alright occasionally however can also cause energetic peaks and valleys, whereas 21 repetitions is more like a steady plateau.

In between each Rite, stand straight with your hands at your hips and your feet together, like Superman, and take two deep breaths. Inhale through your nose and exhale through your mouth with pursed lips, in the shape of an O. Breathe in until around 85% lung capacity and out completely so that every bit of air is exhaled. Imagine inhaling positive energy and exhaling stale air. Imagine further transmutation of the elements into energy though you and the movements.

Begin each movement with inhalation through the nostrils and return on the exhalation. Movement and breath should be slow, steady and performed in unison. The easiest way to count the Rites is saying the number to yourself as you inhale and exhale.

Perform the Rites, Tibetan Fusion, or any yoga, tai chi, chi gung at any time, but most preferably in the morning, when the world is quiet, on an empty stomach. Use a mat or blanket.

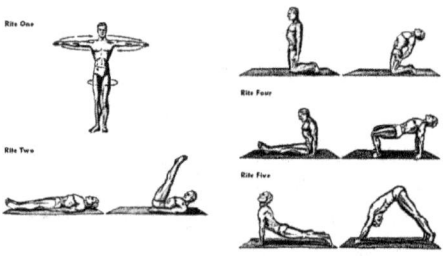

Rite One: spin clockwise with your hands active, palms facing down. The slower you perform each Rite the better access to energy and the more physical the workout as you fight gravity for longer periods of time. Spin clockwise in coordination with breath, inhaling on the first 180 degrees rotation, exhaling on the second 180 degrees of the rotation. Go slow. A variation to lessen exertion is to hold your forearms up at 90 degrees, palms facing inward and spin in coordination with the breath. This is occasionally done while looking to the right hand, sometimes not. Mostly I move almost excruciatingly slowly with the breath and I always face straight ahead throughout.

Rite one is done clockwise only, as opposed to many meditative movements requiring moving both ways so as to remain balanced. It is done this way because the chakras spin in that direction and the sun moves in this way, the micro reflects the macro. To heighten awareness and increase the difficulty of Rite one try integrating the pa qua practice called walking the square. One can walk 360 degrees in four steps by bringing the heel to make contact with the toes and then the other heel to the toe in alternating rotational steps. The walk literally creates a small square in your steps. This brings awareness and attention to the feet and increases the mind body connection and is simply a refinement that can be integrated to raise awareness. Tai chi theory states basically that when we bring awareness to our feet it helps bring awareness to the posture of our entire body.

Take the two deep breaths as described on completing 21 or your set.

Rite Two: lie down flat on your back with the palms down at your sides. Think about keeping your tailbone on the ground as you move. Try to lift up and set down your neck and legs at the same time this helps keep the tailbone on the ground. On the inhalation you rise and on the exhalation you return your neck, shoulders and legs to the floor slowly and gently. Keep the sides of your feet touching. All these positions should be done with straightness in mind, however do not lock your joints —ever, during any movement. If you can lift your legs slightly past ninety degrees do so, but ninety or approaching ninety degrees is adequate. It's actually easier to go to ninety degrees or just beyond. This movement and the following Rites are originated in, open up and power up the abdominal and neck regions. Imagine the breath, the inhalation creates the movement upward.

Tai chi and chi gung principles insist one not strain oneself during stretching and treat it as just being in a position. Yoga practices often seek to settle farther and deeper. The Rites can be a strain, but you should not endure pain. Do them as best you can, as many as you can. Strain the Rites is alright, pain is not. Treat the Rites or any such practice as a walk. One does not have to traverse the valley perfectly, without stepping in one puddle or stumbling on one rock and one can still arrive at your destination on time.

Rite Two prepares the body for Rite Three. The abdominal and neck movement dynamics are opposite. Rite Three transitions to Four and Four is basically the opposite of and preparatory for Five. Don't forget to rise to your feet to take two breaths. Shift to the right side and gently rise to your feet, or do any variation of squats or if you are feeling limber in a gentle yet swiftly in the final movement. Bring your hands above your head and lift your legs up so the knees are bent and the feet arise up off the floor as well as the lower back then rock onto your feet and to standing position.

Rite Three: set your knees about four inches apart and settle on your knees and your toes also four inches apart. Keep your hands just under your buttock with your thumbs slightly grasping the sides of your legs. Use your hands to support your movement and try to keep the elbows from pointing outward extremely. Bend back gently never straining to the point of pain. When you return to starting position on the exhalation return far enough so that you back is straightened. Initially requiring you bend slightly forward past 90 degrees in order to straighten out the back in this position. Keep your shoulders active, but loose.

Each Rite can be seen as opposing the other in an abdominal dynamic, as opening us up. After Rite Three I occasionally like to fold forward onto my palms, so I'm on my hands and knees, hands below shoulders, knees below under my hips. Inhale, look up and bend your back, then exhale looking downward and arch out the back. This can be done two or three times.

Remember to take two breaths in between each Rite. Inhaling through the nose and exhaling through the mouth.

Rite Four: set your hands at the side or your hips your palms facing forward, keep your arms straight and your ankles about four inches apart. Keep your ankles and hands in place —unless you need to adjust. This is often the most difficult Rite to master for most. The main initial mistake is moving one's shoulders and arms. Keep them straight in alignment with your back and at your hips. Inhale from there to a table without moving. As intense as this movement can be on the arms remember to utilize your abdominal strength.

Take two breaths with your hands at your hips.

Rite Five: set your hands and feet at the same width, shoulder width or just a little wider than shoulder width, keep arms and legs in line and in place —unless you need to adjust, as you go. Think about keeping your knees and elbows unlocked. Remain on your toes/balls of your feet and palms throughout the entire movement. Begin in the cobra variation position and inhale to downward dog. Then exhale from upside down V or downward dog back into cobra position. Remember that after the Fourth Rite your muscles are ready to fire off in the opposing movement of the fifth Rite. Move slowly with the breath and maintain a light bend in your knees and elbows without forcefully locking them.

As you progress you can bend your elbows more and more moving downward so that your nose brushes by the floor in a slight swoop a lot like a snake or cobra with your face sliding just above the ground on the exhale and then rise up to the completed position looking upward doing what many call a Hindi pushup. The more you unlock or bend your elbows the deeper work the position affords.

When complete stand up and take the two breaths. Shake it off, ring the bell or walk around a but before lying down to meditate or integrating this bandha, often called the sixth Tibetan.

Add the Sixth Rite when you can do 21 repetitions of each, if you are able. Begin with just one of the Sixth Rite and increase to 3-5. The Sixth Rite should only be included after at least a few days of practicing the Five Tibetan Rites with all 21 repetitions and is not necessary. The Sixth Tibetan raises sexual energy levels for transmutation into life energy and is only done a few times as opposed to the others. 21 repetitions of the Five Rites, plus the Sixth Rite done 3 times equates to 108 movements. I find 2 repetitions in not enough and 4 can be too much, making 3 ideal.

Remaining celibate or withholding ejaculation for at least a couple of days, the longer the better, can enhance one's vitality. Practicing the Five Rites of Rejuvenation, to where you can remember their order and can perform the full 21 repetitions can assist transmutation of sexual energy into life energy by then including the Sixth Rite of Rejuvenation. It is the only Rite that should be done no more than four or five times, three being plenty. Celibacy or withholding ejaculation is not absolutely necessary in order to perform the Sixth Rite, but can enhance its power. In yoga traditions and sense control is one of the eight limbs of yoga and in chi gung it's often called reversing the water or flow. Such bandhas, like the breath control of the sixth Tibetan enhance transmutation.

The sixth Tibetan is extremely powerful bandha or energy lock, and should be treated as such. Begin in the same position as in the two breaths in between each Rite, hands at hips, feet about four inches or so apart. Inhale deeply and then exhale completely, to the point the diaphragm is contracted as you reach for your knees looking downward. Keep a slight arch in the back. Willfully exhale totally and completely through your mouth to the point your abdomen contracts tightly and you contain basically zero breath. Then rise back up the starting position used in between each Rite without inhaling and maintaining abdominal contraction. Do not inhale on the rise up and hold your breath as long as you can comfortably while maintaining slightly tucked chin. A Chinese expression on holding the breath is to do so as long as one can without making yourself angry. And inhale after not holding too long as you lift your chin imagining a rush of balanced energy.

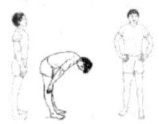

As you practice the Five Rites you might find you want to do more than 21 repetitions so as to get that same physical rush when 21 repetitions required more exertion. Doing more than 21 say 24 or 27 repetitions made me feel dynamic and open, but often resulted in energy swings. It's not necessary to do more than 21 to get the chakras spinning optimally.

The best thing to do is perform them more slowly and be more mindful of your movement, your steps, your neck, your footing, you fingers and all the minute movements. For more of a workout perform them all super slowly, press down on your palms and forearms on #2, go farther on #3, bend elbows more on #4, go lower with elbows bent more on #5 and hold your breath longer #6. You can also do the entire Five Rites in 115 breaths and no more until you take a breather before doing #6.

If the Five Tibetans are all too difficult for you currently, because of an injury or another imbalance utilize the following variations to build on your health and ability. For Rite #1 ring the bell or rotate the axis for 21 breaths. For Rite #2 lie on your back and forearms with head up and then lift your torso so your weight is resting on your forearms and you're looking ahead. Then lift your legs up however much you can on the inhale and back down on the exhale reaching for 21 repetitions. For Rite #3 try to go into the same position and just try to look up 21 times in the same manner as described without pressure on lower back. If your leg is hurt and you simply cannot be in this position yet try lying on your stomach, legs and balls of the feet however and lifting your neck and head upward with and then down to slightly rest on the forehead, with your hands about under your shoulders. For rite #4 lie flat on your back with your arms at your sides with your knees bent and ankles toward your buttock. From this position lift your lower back up and set back down 21 times. For Rite #5 set yourself on your knees (under hips) and palms (under shoulders) with your feet set straight behind you on the balls of the feet. Inhale to downward dog, to upside down V position with knees and elbows unlocked. Aim to set your ankles on the floor and return to starting position on exhale 21 times. Perform the variation of the Rites with the same breaths in between, mindful of performing each Rite the same number of times in coordination with the breath and soon you will be able to do the original Five Rites.

Side note on Rites: I've often been asked why 21 repetitions. The short answer is, I don't know. Maybe because the set approaches 108, but it definitely feels like the optimal number as far as the aforementioned energy plateau. However there are 21 forms of Tara, the Tibetan Buddhism feminine archetype, the Green Tara being the most often venerated. As the story goes there were 20 caves of the Tibetan Saint Milarepa, plus his own cave or house, that of his consciousness, making 21. There are also 21,000 corruptions of ignorance, passion, hatred and a mixture making a total of 84,000 corruptions or Skandas on this plane of existence. Buddha offered 84,000 lessons or dharmas to counter them, of course. Recently it came to be commonly accepted that to repeat a movement 21 times is to memorize it and rub it into muscle memory if you will. Each of these contains possible relationships, but it seems 21 is optimal just because of how it feels more than anything.

There are many questions about the Five Rites. What is certain is they work and they seemingly originated in a place where everything is based on spirit and everything is sacred. Many things about the Rites are mysterious, but the fact that the total number of movements approaches and sometimes is exactly 108 movements, leads me to think of a Pentagon because within pentagons each corner is 108 degrees. When I think of pentagons I think about other triangular patterns and there is something stunning to be said in regards to that.

I think the movements correlate the pyramidal idea in a Merkabah, of two intersecting spinning pyramids. Merkahbah is translated to counter rotational light body vehicle. Think of that translation and the movements of the Rites when you do them. The first movement begins the rotational aspects, the second movement presents a triangle pointing upwards, the third movement is a fluctuating triangular shape, the fourth movement goes from triangular to square, and the fifth goes from triangular to complete triangle. The vortex spinning occurs within you, and around you when the Rites are done frequently as the very movements themselves suggest.

21. Meditate. Follow up the Five Rites of Rejuvenation, accompanied by Sixth only if you can do 21 repetitions of each 5, with meditation. Lay down flat on your back, with your palms facing up just at your sides. One trick in pursuing meditation is to focus on the breath. Breathe through your nose and think of only the tip of your nose. Imagine relaxing so much your body settles into the floor, the only part of your body activated are the tips of your fingers so as to keep you palms flat and settled down too. The longer you meditate after The Five Rites or any meditative movement the more you benefit.

Meditate in the corpse position, the longer being the better. Remember as difficult as many of the movements are, the most difficult part is often mediation. The longer you meditate after doing any of these movements together or separate the more energy will be stirred in the long run. When your energy rises to a certain point you will literally experience bubbling up energy or movement within you that you might have never experienced before. To close meditation reactivate your physical by wiggling your fingers and toes. After meditating in corpse position come up easy by rolling over on your right side, with your hands above your head and pushing up as slowly as you like. Finally meditate a little more sitting cross legged, if you have the time, the longer the better.

Meditation and a meditative mind state is the pinnacle purpose of all yoga, chi gung, tai chi and any like internal art. All such practices operate in a progression toward a meditative mind through movement and all practices end in meditation for meditation is the very point, each and every time you practice and of a practice in total. The longer you meditate afterwards The Five Rites of Rejuvenation or any meditative movements the more you benefit. Movement results in balance, balance provides opportunity for centering, enabling optimal conditions for healing and wellness.

Include chanting the mantra 'Om mani padme hum' when you meditate. Say it aloud in your deepest voice and in your head or just in your head while contemplating its meaning. This simple six syllable phrase is one of praise and compassion and is itself praised in Tibet. Learning the meaning of this mantra is like learning simple meditative movement, it's easy to understand the concept, but its vastness always increases. Just the first syllable Om is alone a window of ideas so amazing that it can be used on its own as a mantra. Simply chanting 'Om' all alone in a deep voice can resonate powerful energy. Om is the eternal hum of the universe known as the unstruck sound. It symbolizes god energy and consciousness. 'Mani' means jewel and 'Padme' means lotus flower, together meaning jeweled lotus flower. The jeweled lotus flower symbolizes our ability to connect with compassionate wisdom. Hum signifies the indivisible aspects of method and practice and the permanent seed of the infinite within the finite. There are countless layers to this welcoming mantra, but a simple way to look at it is as if you are part of a chorus of practitioners chanting in connection with the consciousness of the jeweled lotus flower seed of life.

When you're finished meditating, wiggle your toes and fingers and then begin to move your legs and arms and gently rise by rolling over to the right side first. Sit up and lastly stimulate the bubbling wells. This is a highly beneficial activity to cap off meditative movement of any sort. Rub the soles of your feet 81 times -or more- with the knife edge of you hand, that is the pinky side of the hand. You can do this once, twice or many times a day, at any time. 81 times is the minimum one should rub one's soles, 81 being three fourths of 108 and containing the 1 and the 8 and equating to 9. Rubbing the soles 108 times is definitely just as good and possibly better than 81 times. 81 times is the minimum number one should rub your feet in this way in order to attain benefits. This rubbing technique is separate from the rest of the bone tapping series because it is so powerful on it's on and as an ending movement, but can be integrated with bone tapping the rest of the bod, it can be done by itself whenever.

In Chinese and Ayurvedic medicine the soles of the feet are essentially microcosmic reflections of the rest of the body where all meridian lines reflect reflexology, so when we stimulate the feet, we stimulate the whole body. Some of the most important and most overlooked energy points or chakras are just behind the ball of the feet, sometimes called the bubbling spring wells. The chi gung massage is said to alone yield to good health and longevity through stimulation of this point just behind the ball of the foot. Do not try to look for the chakra, or be exact, simply allow the knife edge of your hand to set into the shape of the sole of the foot, at a slight angle as it naturally fits and rub as a saw. Imagine stimulating the rooting power of the bubbling spring well.

Stimulation of chakra points is a big part of building inner energy, imagine a Tibetan singing bowl. These chakra points are metaphysical points in the body which link the physical and spiritual. During meditative movement these aspects are brought together via the invigoration of these points. When finished meditate in a siting posture or rise up lightly and walk it off.

Try bathing or showering before doing any energy work, but do not bathe or shower directly afterward doing meditative movement. It's recommended universally to wait fifteen minutes at least.

As you begin to master yourself and experience energy it's likely you are going to want to learn more tai chi, chi gung and yoga. A few moves you can immediately integrate into your asana set are shoulder stands, the plow pose and even a simple head stand. These require further tutelage, I believe, but a basic outline for each is below for those with experience.

The plow essentially starts lying down on your back. Bring with your feet up and over you head so your toes reach behind your head aiming to have your knees straight, but unlocked so that you are resting on your back, neck and toes behind your head. This is a tremendous move, take a class if you do not have experience. To do a shoulder begin in the same position. Think about being gentle and symmetrical. Knees remain bent and then with a bit of rocking power bring legs above your head and shift yourself so that you palms are on your lower back and forearms are on the floor as stabilization. Bring your legs straight up so they are pointed up with your feet relaxed forward so your toes are straight up from your gaze. Hold this position for a breath or two and as you become more comfortable numerous breaths. If you feel you might fall, maybe wait then.

The easiest headstand is performed by simply transforming the crow posture. The crow is done pressing the palms of your hands onto the floor and then pressing your knees behind your bent forearms. Lift your legs so that you are balancing all your weight on your hands knees pressing into forearms. Begin the headstand by pressing palms into the floor with your legs behind you, knees resting on arms. Slowly press your head into the floor, then bring your knees to behind your forearms and finally lift your toes off the ground balancing on your hands and head, knees pressing behind your bent forearms. You can remain in this position, or raise your feet straight upward, really pressing through the fingertips, Place a blanket underneath your head if you find the firmness uncomfortable. I suggest integrating these asanas into your asana sets as you feel comfortable, toward the end.

For further headstands you need an instructor as well as for handstands though you can practice building your strength using a wall to prop your feet on for balance. With your back to the wall press your palms on the floor about two and half or three feet from the wall. Press your body weight onto your palms and begin walking up the wall. When you are now standing on your hands you can walk balk, on your hands, to the wall a bit more. Remain there for ten seconds or a minute or more. To exit that position walk forward with your hands and down with your feet. Seek instruction for more.

On Walking

After practicing Tibetan Fusion don't just sit down and relax –unless your work involves such. Integrate your yogi mind, your chi power and do something positive for yourself and the world. And walk lightly when doing so. Walk lightly for long life.

Notice how people walk, where they put and shift their weight, how heavily they step and at what angles they point their feet. And pay attention to how you stand and walk. Martial artists seek to have heavy hands, to have heavy hands one must be relaxed like a baby and throw your weight uninhibitedly. Alternatively they seek to be light on their feet. Unhealthy people tend to walk heavily, stomping and flopping their weight through their hips or knees, pronating their lower backs, whereas healthy people tend to walk softly sending their weight to the balls of their feet. When you walk think about your light feet. Think about your footing, it's said when you are mindful of your feet you become mindful of your whole body.

Pa qua, the art from which walking the square originates, is a kung fu practice in which many of the training methods and forms involve walking in a circle and performing turns, twists, strikes and holding prone positions. The circular walking is done slowly and rapidly too. Walking in a circle and perhaps even more so spinning in a circle creates a vortex, but also develops balance and strength when done as part of pa qua. In the old schools practitioners would walk in circles for many months, perfecting their footwork before learning forms, the circle walking is the 20% of pa qua supplying 80% of the benefit. One of the forms in pa qua is called the teacup form. The teacups form is one of the most dynamic and yet simple movements that like all of pa qua can be used and done many ways. Just like the first movement of the Five Tibetan Rites pa qua can frequently involve simply standing and spinning. The martial application of spinning makes it essentially so that one cannot be grabbed or easily confronted for unpredictable elbows, fists, knees and kicks are constantly being thrown and twisting steps are constantly creating confusing motion. The energetic understanding is that spinning, as well as circle walking, creates and stimulates vortexes in and around the body, symbolized by the chakra points and our aura or energy field surrounding us.

Imagine holding teacups in your palms so your hands face up during the entire form. Your hands, with bent elbows and relaxed shoulders, make a swirl in the form of an infinity symbol. Start standing with your feet a little wider than shoulder width apart, knees bent, hips open. Raise your left hand above you head, with palms up so that your forearm, near your wrist, just brushes above and behind your head. Twist the arm around and out so your hand and fingers are pointing away from you, elbow nearly extended, then swirl your hand back across chest toward opposite side and curl back across and down continuing along so that your left hand then goes behind your left hip. Then swirl hand in front of you and back up to the starting position, with the elbow bent, brushing your head. Do so in one slow graceful movement.

When one has figured out this movement integrate both hands. Then integrate moving the body so that the hands are but an extension of the body movement beginning with movement from the lower abdominals or dantien. Begin by bending, twisting and flowing with the hand movements and gradually make the hand movements from the bending and twisting. Perform the hand movements in synchronicity as well as in alternation, moving in unison as well as one hand being high while the other is low. When done in alternation he tea cups form ends up looking a lot like Neo in The Matrix in the famous scene where he dodges bullets, only without the special effects.

And when you have figured out doing it with both hands, integrate spinning in place. Then perform teacups, spinning, while walking in a circle. The tea cups form as a walking meditation has it all; back bends, forward folds, twists, spins, shoulder and arm loosening, balance practice and mind/body integration. The martial applications work as the various movements can transform into locks, strikes, twisting combinations and blocks, but the energetic applications are always accessible no matter. Perform the teacups vortex walking slowly. Soon enough you will feel the spiraling energy make you want to speed the form up. It's alright to do so, but the longer you move slow the better.

There are several other walking meditations and other ways to walk so as to change your physical disposition. If you experience lower back, hip, knee or leg pain try walking like a pigeon.

Li Ching Yun, potentially the longest lived person advised to, "Keep a quiet heart, sit like a tortoise, walk sprightly like a pigeon and sleep like a dog." Stay calm and compassionate, sit still and meditate, walk lightly with toes slightly pointed inward (at least occasionally) and go to sleep early and rise up early.

Walking like a pigeon immediately straightens your back, betters your posture and makes you mindful of your body from the feet up. It also makes all the sinews in the hips and lower back readjust after years of not being mindful of your feet. Instead of unthinkingly setting ourselves in a way our toes are always pointed out we turn them inward adjusting our whole body. It's a beneficial position on its own and it's a change. Sometimes simply a change is enough of a reset to help heal, even if only done occasionally. You can also try walking with just one foot pigeon toed and the other set normally. We spend so much time standing and walking pronated that this change can be tremendously healing.

Try walking by setting your toes down first instead of your heels, dos walking slowly. Again it's just a change, resulting in lessening of old strains and awareness from the feet up.

Walk extremely slowly. Walk in coordination with slow and relaxed breath.

Walk while ringing the bell. Step forward slowly as you ring the bell softly and gently.

Learn to perform the tai chi walk or cat crawl which is essentially walking and performing open hand strike. Step forward with right and strike with left, step forward with left and strike with right. One should sweep with the hand and arm that is not striking so that for a moment during shift next strike it is as if you are holding a ball of energy. The tai chi walk can be done walking backwards too. In the same way step with one foot and strike with the opposite hand. Remember to try to meditate while walking and be meditative as you go about your business. A trick to do this is by focusing on being in your head as if a single point in the middle of your head behind what people point to as the third eye chakra and imagine as if you're walking on clouds.

Alternatively try walking imagining you are in a field of thick mud. Another related idea is to imagine that as you go you weigh 10,000 pounds as you go and you're feet are so heavy that no matter your strength they move slowly. When doing so move slowly and don't slam your feet to the floor of course.

Tibetans walk, climb and traverse great distances in the mountainous region where the air is thin, at an altitude where one tends to feel heavier and weighed down. A legendary walking meditation was utilized by Tibetan Buddhists to travel great distances in short periods. It is known as the practice of lung gum. Lung means wind/air energy or chi/prana and gum means meditation. This form of meditational walking or running is said to enhance speed, balance, climbing agility and overall ability to make passage through the rugged mountains. Some people were known to be so light footed and fast that from a distance it appeared they were an approaching quadruped.

Lung gum involves a secret acrobatic breathing technique using internal air. The practice somehow overcomes the normal limitations in obtaining oxygen for our moving muscles. It is not a sprinters trick for short moments of high speed running, but an untiring high speed gate which legend states can turn a month long journey into a two day trip, running the entire time.

In order to experience lung gum chant the mantra, 'Om mani padme hum' or 'lung gum pa' (pa addition means practitioner) as you proceed. You can say the mantra aloud for a bit, but then just say it to yourself. Try to focus on the mantra and then allow yourself to focus on breathing. Meditate on being full of light and light footed. Your steps should be as one who bounces forward. Your presence should be as if a single point in the center of your head. Your focus should be in the distance.

In order to experience lung gum one must silence the mind and be in the now. The components may seem like a lot to contemplate, but eventually the muscle memory takes over the meditation, just as muscle memory takes over running, so one can eventually just be mindful of one thing; the breath and then completely in the moment, the mind thinking nothing, the consciousness in the now.

Part of the lung gum tradition is to have an eternal stare into the distance utilizing a peripheral vision stare as you go. This assists in being in that open and relaxed mind state where the mind is quiet and consciousness is in the now. One should fix one's attention ahead and just slightly upward according to tradition as if looking at a star on the horizon. Many people can experience lung gum, just as many people can experience Tummo, however to become proficient takes devoted refinement of the meditative mind. Run as if carried. Move as if light. Bounce as you go along in a mantra trance and imagine yourself a consciousness vehicle designed to cover great distances. Imagine a time when you possessed the undefeatable resolution of a child with new shoes and newfound speed.

We are all equally capable of walking and meditation. Both make one more capable and more healthful overall. Walking and meditating are similar in that they are good for us in many ways and connect us in many ways. The next time you're walking or the next time walking seems mundane, a simple physical process, imagine Buddha or Jesus or whoever you look up to walking as you, then the process become metaphysical. Many yogis and Buddha himself, according to legend left their footprints in granite as it were mud. When the process of walking or whatever it may be seems merely physical remember to contemplate the mental, spiritual, and universal aspects of what you're doing as well to make it all metaphysical.

The practice of lung gum is one of the most refined forms of meditative running or jogging to cover long distances, just as many of the meditations from Tibet are some of the most refined and effective cover long distances within. Many cultures have similar walking meditations as well as standing, lying and sitting meditations, whether called meditations or simply interpretable as meditative movement, called dances or noted as some other form of ritualistic circle walking.

The Buddhist monks in Japan on Mt. Hiei share a similarly amazingly developed running or walking meditation to the Tibetan practice of lung gum, though it is probably more demanding and exact. The marathon monks or running monks as they are commonly referred to have the most famous and arduous running traditions. They practice the same type of long distance running with the same type of fixed, undistracted, eternal stare, as if looking at a star ahead.

The most difficult test in this system is a period of nine days or two-hundred and sixteen hours of fasting while running. Many Native American tribes once had customary running rites as did many African cultures. The function of walking and running is part of certain cultural rites and traditions from all across the world. Meditation is the same as walking in this way, variously celebrated and developed the same, albeit in different mannerisms. To begin any journey, physical or meditational, all you have to do is put one foot in front of the other.

~Please leave a review for Tibetan Fusion. Read Ethan Indigo Smith's similar works 108 Steps to Be in The Zone and The Matrix of Four The Philosophy of The Duality of Polarity, and The Geometry of Energy How to Meditate.

www.ingramcontent.com/pod-product-compliance
Lightning Source LLC
Chambersburg PA
CBHW070605290526
45790CB00002B/789